Learning by Accident

D0900562

a memoir by
Rosemary Rawlins

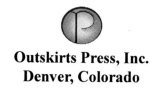

Outskirts Press, Inc.
Denver, Colorado

Outskirts Press, Inc.
http://www.outskirtspress.com

ISBN: 978-1-4327-7325-0

Library of Congress Control Number: 2011926899

Outskirts Press and the "OP" logo are trademarks belonging to Outskirts Press, Inc.

PRINTED IN THE UNITED STATES OF AMERICA

Author's Note:

This book is my confession.

Everyone said I was strong and brave when I cared for my husband as he recovered from a traumatic brain injury. But I was the cowardly lion who wanted to turn and run from the wizard's booming voice across the room that declared the end of my life as I knew it.

Until one day I asked myself, what is bravery? And a small voice (not what you'd expect—you'd expect a very big voice from bravery) said: bravery is simply taking a tentative step, then another, until you are walking— through puddles, deep trenches, and mud—till you reach the other side, and you're running.

Dedicated to:

Hugh, for teaching me life lessons every day, and for giving me two extraordinary daughters.

...and to my mother, for showing me caregiving at its best.

In recognition:

of all the caregivers who work tirelessly to help loved ones, sometimes losing and always rearranging their own lives in the process. May you find strength in the joy of the selfless act, the gift inherent in giving, and the peace that comes from doing the right thing.

Foreword

As a medical professional, I have been called upon many times over the past 30 years to care for patients with severe head injuries. Little did I know that while I was caring for the patient described in this book, Hugh Rawlins, that his clinical course and experience, and that of his family would be so compassionately, realistically, and humanly depicted in this book.

As health professionals, we often concentrate on the science of caring for the patient and forget the human and emotional toll that it takes on patients, their families, and surrounding friends. This book describes in a touching, yet authentic manner, the effect that severe head injury can have on a patient, as well as his family and friends. In my reading of this book, I found a new and expanded appreciation of what patients and families experience during this time of medical crisis.

Mrs. Rawlins has done the medical profession, especially those who treat head injury, a great service by her warm and detailed description of her and her husband's journey. I feel privileged to have been asked to write this foreword, and I feel privileged to have been involved in Mr. Rawlins' care.

John D. Ward, M.D., MSHA
Hirschler Professor & Vice Chair
Department of Neurosurgery
Co-Director, Harold F. Young Neurosurgical Center

Acknowledgements

I owe my deepest gratitude and love to Hugh, Anna, and Mary for allowing me to write about their lives in such a personal way. Hugh, thank you for loving me, you are my safe place. Mary and Anna, you make me shine. I love you the *infinitiest!*

Thank you, Mom and Pop, I miss you every day. Warmest thanks to my brothers and sisters and their husbands and wives: Peg & Toni (for reading and editing), Bill & Cindy, John & Sue, Pat & Jim, and Mary & Dan. I am so blessed to have you all in my life. Thank you, Lisa Kron, for your beautiful words.

Special thanks to my mother-in-law and father-in-law, Rita and Hugh Rawlins, for being there every step of the way, and for helping to make this book possible. Thank you, Betty, David, and Krista O'Connell for your helping hands, loving notes, and visits.

Every girl needs great girlfriends, and mine are the best. For pep talks, sharing laughter and tears, long walks, gifts, meals, music, visits, and magical massages…Thank you: Terry Cleveland, Patty King, Peggy Thibodeau, Electra Liatos, Nancy Tomlinson, Kelly King, Celeste Young, Debbie Willis, KiKi Nusbaumer, Terry Little, and Lara Meili. Words cannot express how much I love you.

Thank you, Leane Elliott, for stopping at the accident scene and keeping Hugh safe until help arrived; and to Wray Eldridge, our brave witness. Thank you, Ed Wood, and the nine firemen of Station 15 who rescued Hugh and rushed him to MCV. You did everything right that day and we will never forget you.

My heartfelt thanks go to Dr. John Ward for his surgical genius, and for always telling us that healing does not stop after three months, six months, or a year…but continues on. We believed you and it mattered. Our gratitude extends to MCV Hospital, and its extraordinary nurses and residents, particularly Dr. Jason Highsmith, Charlotte Gilman and Kathy McCurdy; and with love to Barbara Farley for helping me feel at home in a hospital, for beautiful lunches out and dinners she brought in. Thank you!

Thank you HealthSouth: Dr. Roger Giordano, Nancy Foley, Penny Eissenberg, Jennifer Floyd, Michaelle Justice, and Cathy Satterfield for providing outstanding care and therapy, compassionate counseling, and amazing skill.

Thank you Dr. Jeff Kreutzer for helping us create a new life, one that we love.

Thank you Evonne, our beloved night sitter.

Thank you Jason Blake, for your friendship, expertise and athletic coaching.

With deep gratitude and love for The Church of the Epiphany, our spiritual home. Special thanks to the Rev. Dr. Keith Emerson, Diana Stone (who visited the hospital every day), and all who brought meals, visited, and prayed for us. All prayers were deeply felt.

Deepest thanks to Lee and Barbara Facetti for your unfailing friendship, campy jokes, filing our taxes, driving us around, and helping Hugh get back to work.

Thanks to the cycling gang: Kevin Dintino, Jim Eicher, Rick Meili, and Fred Allyn for physical therapy help, yard work, driving, and inspirational visits. Thank you Donnelle Dintino for your friendship.

Thank you, Lee Piper, for attending Hugh's team meeting with me and for your advice and encouragement.

Many thanks to Liz and Ken West. Liz, your legal expertise was much appreciated.

Deepest thanks to Ed and Margaret Martin for your prayers, helping hands and generosity of spirit.

Thank you, Lawrence Liesfeld for your southern hospitality and willingness to help.

Thank you Tom, Brett, Michelle, Dixie and all of Hugh's wonderful coworkers who sent us beautiful notes, gift baskets, and visited us during Hugh's recuperation.

Thank you Bambi and Harley Jones for being two of the most beautiful women I know—and for the daily gifts of love you sent to our front door for weeks on end.

Many thanks to my large Irish family, the Healey and Flaherty clans, especially cousins: Jim Flaherty, Larry and Angela McNaughton, KiKi Burpee, Peter McNaughton, and Rich Flaherty.

Thank you Greg and Celie Florence for your friendship, and your healing gift of the beach—including all those meals at Chez Flo's!

Thank you to our neighbors: Chris and Tom Duggins, Scott and Theresa Pelais, Tim and Jennifer Tabler, and Bernadette for the delicious meals you sent.

Special thanks to my sister, Pat Waters, and my niece, Emma, for designing the beautiful cover of my book, and Nancy Tomlinson for taking the cover photo.

Very special thanks to Jan Tarasovic. Without you, Jan, I would not have published this book. Your initial response, careful editing, and constant encouragement reignited my energy and made me believe I could do this.

…and to my writer's group, John Bruns, Don Warner, David Thomas and the late Paul Brandt—thank you for reading and rereading passages and blurbs until I'm sure you were quite tired of the story—but never said so.

Thank you everyone that helped us out in big and small ways. As Bambi Jones says, "We are spiritually bound—all of us on this earth." Your kindness will never be forgotten.

Chapter 1

Hugh's mind spins as quickly as the blurred spokes on the wheels of his bike. He pedals through a clear spring afternoon on the last leg of a twenty-mile route he has ridden for over ten years: Springfield to Nuckols Road, right on Shady Grove, and into the Virginia countryside before winding around on Pouncy Tract by Rockville School. He's determined to get back in shape. Logging far too many hours in the office during winter has taken its toll. The burning in his quads reminds him to get out more so he can rejoin the rigorous Saturday morning group ride he enjoys. Vowing to whip himself into shape in two weeks, he smiles inwardly, his mood elevated by the wind cooling his face as he quickens his pace. Dressed in full gear, he glides along, feeling the stress of the workweek evaporate as quickly as the sweat pouring down his face.

He hears a car. Before he can glance over his shoulder, his head snaps back, both hands fly off the handlebars as the bike is ripped out from under him. He feels his toe clips release. He feels his body slide across the metal hood and smash into the windshield. Glass shatters into a million sparkling beads that bounce around him like a meteor shower. Tossed upward into an awkward flight, he shoots over the car roof glimpsing blurred images of earth, sky, a truck, and treetops, until an earsplitting clunk sends blades of pain ripping across his forehead. His thick bike helmet cracks. Writhing in shock, he sprawls on the street, his skin scraped off in road-burned sections. His eyes close and open. One-word thoughts stab him into consciousness—blackness…

sunlight...burning...girls.

A young nurse is on her way home from Lowe's with her husband and son. Traffic stalls. Craning their necks, they notice a gathering crowd. "Must be an accident," her husband says, "I'll wait here. You go do what you do best." She pushes her long hair away from her face, throws off her flip-flops and runs. Several distraught people surround the accident victim. As the nurse approaches, she says to two men, "Don't try to move him." A towel roll has been placed under his head. "Has anyone called an ambulance?" she asks.

"I think so," answers a tall young man, voice shaking.

"I'm an R.N.," she says, kneeling. "I'll stay with him." Swallowing hard, she naturally blocks out the sound of cars whizzing by to make her quick assessment: blood and gunk flooding his ears, pupils abnormally dilated. Head injury—acute. The man's eyes widen with unspeakable pain as he tries to talk while kicking his legs on the hard road. "Help me, help me," he grunts. She kneels beside him and takes his pulse. He jerks away. "Leave me alone!" he yells. The nurse's eyes travel up his arm where a chunk of torn flesh flaps on his elbow.

"You've been in an accident. Lie still. Help is coming," she says in the most even voice she can manage. Her face hovers directly over his as their eyes lock in the sunlight.

"I can hear the fire trucks. They're coming to help you. Hang on." She can barely stand to look into his frenzied blue eyes. It's as if they are screaming—pleading with her to understand a message she should deliver. "What is it?" she asks. He turns to his right, screams again in pain, as she spots the gold wedding band on his left hand. She knows instantly that he has a wife who needs to know how badly he's hurt. What if she's at home planting flowers at this very moment? Does he have children? She grips his hand tightly, joined in the horror of his pain and his inability to communicate. She watches the sun reflect the shock in his eyes. "What is your name?" she asks.

He moans low and deep, as if he can't hear her. "Stay calm. Keep still," she soothes. "You'll be fine." Rubbing his arm in long slow strokes, she allows herself to take a deep breath. As an R.N. in the hospital, she has seen injury, but never the raw pain and sheer panic of an accident scene. She knows that with every passing second his life is ebbing away. She watches him grow weaker, more tired, but determined to live. "Stay with me," she says louder when his eyes close. He opens them again, piercing blue reflecting the sky.

Traffic backs up despite the effort of a twenty-year-old desperately directing cars. He checks in now and then with the nurse, his eyes glazed with tears. His tattooed arm directs bystanders to the roadside, forming an audience of paralyzed, whispering witnesses like a retaining wall around the scene.

The shrill siren grows louder and louder until, abruptly, it stops. The nurse hears doors crank open, hurried footsteps. Within seconds, paramedics arrive. As she steps aside to let others take over, the injured man curses and thrashes in a wild burst of energy. It takes nine firemen to strap him to a body board.

Running toward her van, bawling repressed tears, the nurse collapses into her husband's arms. She buries her face in his shirt to drown out the primal shriek of the cyclist as he's lifted onto the stretcher. Who is this man? How can she let go of him and leave him now? When she hears others scrambling in their search to locate some form of I.D. for the cyclist, she breaks away from her husband, runs over to the car that struck the bike, and sees a twisted knot of scrap metal wedged under the front fender. Peering under for clues, she finds none, so she continues to search for a wallet or saddlebag along the pavement. A few feet from the damaged car, she notices a policewoman speaking to a small group of people on the side of the road. An older woman glances over at her, oddly detached. A younger man is crying openly while gesturing to the officer.

Off in a patch of soft grass, someone yells, "Over here!" A cell phone is rushed to a rescue worker who presses *Contacts*, sees the word *home*, and calls the nearest trauma hospital with the number, as the doors to the ambulance slam shut.

The nurse feels a firm hand grip her shoulder, "Ready to go?" asks her husband. She lets her head fall on his shoulder. Minutes ago she was on a happy outing with her family. Now she hears only questions and the shrieks of a dying man in her head.

Chapter 2

I fumble with overstuffed brown bags and keys, stumble in the front door, and hear the phone ring as I dump paper sacks on the kitchen table and grab the phone.

"This is MCV Hospital—do you know a cyclist?" asks an urgent voice.

For a moment I can't speak. The voice shatters my silence, "Hello? Are you there?"

"It's my husband. Is he okay?"

"No. A car hit him. He's in serious condition. You need to come down here."

"How serious? What happened?"

"It would be best if you could just get here right away."

"I'll be there." I hang up and stare at the phone, shaking. I have never been to MCV. I know it's downtown, but two other hospitals are closer. Why the Medical College of Virginia? Instinctively I call a few friends who could take me there, but their answering machines pick up. Just as I hang up on the third call, the phone vibrates and rings loudly in my hand, making me jump before I push the button to answer.

"Hello, this is MCV again; can you give us his name? He had no ID on him."

"Hugh Rawlins, R-A-W-L-I-N-S. How did you know to call me?"

"We found your number on his cell phone. Is he diabetic? He may need blood."

It was Hugh. I was hoping they had the wrong person. Blood?

"No, he's not diabetic. How do I get there? Give me directions from I-64 heading east."

I scribble the directions, stop for a minute and take a deep breath.

After pulling a list of phone numbers out of the junk drawer, I grab my car keys and run out the door. "Just drive. 64 East to Exit 74C, 74C...." I repeat, talking to myself. At a red light, I call Hugh's friend, Kevin, and reach his voicemail. "Kevin, it's Rosemary. I'm on my way to MCV. Hugh has been in an accident. I think it's bad. I don't know if I can do this alone." My voice breaks up. "Please come."

Stuck behind a slow truck, I want to jump out of the car and run the rest of the way. My litany continues in a strained whisper, "Right on Eleventh Street. Right on Clay."

I find a space in the parking deck, jump out of the car, and race to the emergency room, where the full force of dread hits. A security guard steers me to a policewoman in the hall. "Your husband has been hit by a car," she says quietly. "He's in critical condition. He needs surgery. They are x-raying him now. I'm sorry, but can I get some information? I need his full name and a number where I can reach you later."

Bile rises in my throat as I answer her questions. A young woman in a white coat hurries over. "Mrs. Rawlins?" she asks. I nod.

"My name is Karen. I'm here to help you. I'm sorry about your husband." The two escort me to a small, narrow, whitewashed room with a few chairs, a box of tissues and no windows. "Can I get some information? Correct spelling of your name? Your husband's social security, insurance?" she asks.

I numbly take out my I.D. cards and hand them over. "Can I see him?"

"Yes, in just a moment, before he goes up for surgery." *Why, if this is so urgent, does everything feel like slow motion?*

I look at the police officer. "Who hit him? Was that person hurt too?"

"No, he was the only one hurt. I'll be going now. Is it okay if I call you later for more information?" I nod.

Karen takes over. "Would you like to call someone?" she asks.

"No. Not now." I say it slowly as if trying to stop time. My mind is as blank as the bare walls of the room.

A woman comes in and introduces herself as the hospital chaplain. "I'm sorry about your husband, Mrs. Rawlins," she says. "It looks very serious. What religion are you?" Her voice sounds overly calm.

"Episcopalian."

"Can I help in any way? You will be able to see him, but I must tell you, it's a massive head injury. You may want to say goodbye. Be prepared for the worst."

"No. I won't say goodbye!"

Karen hands me a tissue. Her voice is sweet, like a family member. "Is there anyone nearby who can come here to help you? You should have someone with you.

"No," I repeat. "I won't say goodbye."

"Can I get you a drink of water?" I shake my head no.

"Your husband has multiple injuries. But the most serious one is his head injury. He needs surgery now; we will bring him up soon. We'll certainly do everything we can. Come and see him." She gently takes my hand.

"I can't believe this," I whisper as she guides me like a child across the hall. Hugh is lying flat and still on a gurney, the light over him casting a garish glow. People mill around him, but I'm unaware of what they're doing. He looks dead. No, I tell myself, he's just asleep. I walk over to him and lay my hand on his chest in disbelief. He is real—lying on a gurney—about to have surgery. I'm transfixed. Through hot tears, I see his solid frame dressed in colorful cycling clothes as he walked out the door just a few hours ago. We had said the most casual of goodbyes, no kiss, no hug....

Chapter 3

A whiff of alcohol startles me back to the present. Still in disbelief, I lift Hugh's hand, bruised and swollen at the knuckles. His black cycling shorts are torn and his jersey has been removed. His tan muscular thighs are streaked with lines of blood now drying to a dark crust. Gazing at his unconscious face, I lean close to his ear, "Please don't leave me, Hugh Rawlins, don't let go—I don't want you to go. Mary and Anna need you. I love you." Sensing someone nearby, I look up. An orderly nods sympathetically as Hugh is rolled away for surgery. A gentle tug from Karen tells me to follow.

I'm across the hall in the white room again. "Sit here," Karen says. I register short phrases floating off the cloud that cushions my mind against the onslaught of bad news: "Brain surgery…very serious…long operation." My mind and heart bounce racquetballs off each other, the logical and the hysterical colliding.

"Mrs. Rawlins, is there anyone you can call to come sit with you?"

"Not really. My children are at a party. I have no family here. Hugh's parents are in Florida and mine live in New York." Tears stream down my face. I rub them off and wipe my hands on my jeans. "All my brothers and sisters live out of state."

"Don't you have any friends?"

"Yes, but they're out. I already called some on the way over. I'll be alright." I feel small, curled up like a bug against a huge foot pressing down on me.

"Let me give you a moment, I'll be right outside," she says and leaves me to gather myself. I hear faint murmuring as she consults someone.

My mind drifts back to the day and night before it all happened, wondering if I could have changed the course of events by stalling, lingering, or making love to him when he sent me all the right signals. I resurrect and relive every second, every word, impression, and look he gave me in the twenty-four hours before he was hurt. "Stop it!" I tell myself. "What does it matter anyway? It happened. It's done." Still, like a winding newsreel, it replays in my head.

The night before he crashed, all four of us were home. Hugh and I heard the slamming of a door and the muffled stampeding of a carpeted race downstairs before watching Anna half slide, and nearly fall into the hallway with her sister in full pursuit. They had spotted their ride to the eighth grade dance from the upstairs window. "How can two tiny dancers sound like such a herd of elephants?" I whispered to Hugh, making him smile.

Anna skidded by us first, clad in a tight little skirt and fitted shirt, perfect for her thin straight frame. She brushed soft kisses on our cheeks, turned dramatically, opened the front door, and strutted across the green lawn in mock sophistication. Glancing over her shoulder with a wide smile, her blonde curls bouncing, she waved one last time. "We are in *big* trouble," Hugh whispered to me. After hopping on one leg to adjust a flapping shoe strap, Mary followed with a hurried hug. Even while sprinting to catch up to her sister, she moved gracefully in a swirling skirt of violet flowers, her long brown hair cascading down her back. "Stay away from the boys!" Hugh shouted to them, only half joking.

"Sure Dad!" Mary called back, her eyes rolling with innocence and mischief.

"Those girls are growing up way too fast. Too many guys are calling them. Do you know all these kids?" he asked with a serious look, hesitating to close the front door.

"Well I know that one of them said he had a dream that you were chasing him with a chainsaw, so I guess they all know you are an overprotective father!" This brought a sinister smile to Hugh's face.

"They're fourteen year old boys, Hon. How bad can they be?" I said with shrug. His eyebrows shot up as if to say, "Pretty bad!" Hugh stared at the empty spot where the car had turned the corner. "It sure is strange to think of them going to a dance," he mumbled.

"C'mon. Let's go around the block and eat at that little place by Michael's. I don't feel like cooking," I said, nudging him in the waist. At the restaurant, we talked over drinks.

"Do you have any townhouse work to do with Lee this weekend?" I asked.

"No painting or anything, but he called me today to say he saw a few new condos on the market. Trouble is, both of us are too busy with our day jobs to look into new rentals." He wiped buffalo sauce off the corner of his mouth and asked me about the girls' plans.

"A few friends are throwing a surprise birthday party for them at the ice skating rink. They really have no idea, especially since they already celebrated with us. They won't want me to hang around." Hugh's eyes creased sympathetically. Our knees touched under the table in the cramped booth.

"Any new clients this week?" Hugh asked.

"Two: a Capital One analyst and a store manager who works at Talbot's. Her résumé will write itself. I hate to say this, but I'm getting tired of writing résumés. There are only so many ways to say the same thing."

"Hire people, grow the business, or go back to school. You always planned on finishing your degree," Hugh said.

"Oh, I don't know—it's so time-consuming and expensive. When are you and Anna going to start surfing again?"

"Soon, I hope. I need a wetsuit that fits, though." He tapped his stomach and smirked.

"Think Mary will go?" I asked. Hugh finished his Jack Daniels. I savored my red wine. My salad and his burger were plunked down in front of us.

"She'll go if Amanda goes; those two are joined at the hip. It's weird, but she does look more like Mary than Anna does, people have mistaken them for twins instead of best friends. Anyway, I hope Mary tries it again. She's such a great swimmer."

"It's funny because when I took the girls to see *Titanic*, Anna was scared to death and covered her eyes, but Mary was fine, and now it's Mary that's skittish in the water. She told me she hates the jelly fish and not being able to see the bottom, but I think it was that show, *Summer of the Sharks.*"

"She wants that Roxy surfboard, though," Hugh interjected.

"Yeah, and she knows you won't pay for it unless she learns how to ride it."

"I hope she comes. It's more fun with both of them."

As we left the restaurant, Hugh held the door for me like a gentleman. His old world manners charmed me from the start. Once home, I checked our voicemail, and kicked off my shoes. As we flopped onto the couch together, Hugh signaled me with his eyes. "Alone at last," he whispered. His arm tightened around my waist as I picked up the remote and kicked away the throw pillow blocking my feet. In a half-hearted attempt at romance, his hand wandered under my shirt. My squirming told him to stop, so he rested his hand on my hip after a retaliatory squeeze.

"Sorry hon. I have to pick the girls up soon. What do you want to watch?" I asked.

"Anything," he said, breathing against the back of my neck. Within minutes, he nodded off. Just as I felt sleepy, I slipped away, rubbing his humid breath into my shoulder. I closed the door quietly and left to pick up the girls.

Inside the dark van, Mary reported, "There are no tall boys to dance with. The only two tall boys have girlfriends. But we all danced in groups anyway."

"Mom, check this out, a new dance," Anna said as she demonstrated the percolator making us all laugh out loud as she jerked spastically while strapped in her seat belt. Her snorting laugh made us double over.

"Stop it! I'm trying to drive," I yelled still laughing.

Mary cut in, "When we get home, I want to show you the wedding veil I found on the Internet. It's gorgeous, Mom. It's called a mantilla. Wait till you see it!" She has been planning her wedding since she was five years old.

"Which one is this, Mary? Veil number ten already?"

"No, honest, this is the one," she said earnestly.

Saturday morning, Hugh left early to mow his parents' lawn not far from our house since they were not back from their winter stay in

Florida. I threw a load of laundry in the washer and heard Mary call down the hallway, "Can you buy Snuggles, Mom? Amanda's mom uses Snuggles and it smells so good!" Back in the kitchen, I stole a minute to look at the newspaper while the girls got ready for Skate Nation. The sound of the upstairs shower and calls from room to room told me they were choosing outfits and heaping the floor with wet towels and abandoned clothes as they dressed for their afternoon out.

Hugh returned around lunchtime to grab a sandwich. "How does this look, Dad?" Mary asked him. She stood with her hands on her hips to show off a new shirt. Without looking at her, he mumbled, "You always look beautiful, honey." Grunting audibly, she huffed past him back to her full-length mirror.

"Did I say something wrong?" Hugh whispered to me in a baffled tone. I cocked my head and shrugged. He retreated upstairs to change his clothes and rejoined me in the kitchen.

"What do you want to do tonight?" I asked.

"How about *Training Day* with Denzel Washington," he said, clomping on the kitchen floor in his cycling shoes. He stopped to fill his water bottle at the sink and added, "I'm going for a short ride. I'll be back soon to mow our lawn." He looked like a Times Square billboard in his multicolored cycling jersey against the plain white walls and natural cabinets of our kitchen that some liken to a bowling alley. The girls asked us not to install a breakfast bar so they could practice their dance turns.

I swiped away small crumb pyramids from the table, stacked dirty dishes, and headed toward the sink in my usual clean up mode. "Okay, I'm dropping the girls at Skate Nation. I'll pick up the movie at Blockbuster and meet you back here." Hugh strode to the garage for his bike. "Bye!" he yelled, and the door slammed before I could answer. Up to my elbows in hot bubbly water, I wondered again what was keeping me from going back to school.

While driving the girls to the skating rink, I kept quiet, careful not to ruin the surprise for them. Instead, I wrote a grocery list in my head.

"Pick us up at ten, Mom?" Mary asked as we pulled into the parking lot.

"Hey, can't I even come in for a minute?"

"If you want," Anna said hesitantly. I walked into the lobby with them and saw their delighted faces as friends yelled, "Surprise!" After a quick kiss, I discreetly slipped out as they stood by the sheet cake and stack of gifts. One grocery list later, I stepped into the house clutching brown bags of food. The phone rang, and a voice tore my life out from under me with one question.

"Do you know a cyclist?"

The words reverberate as I sit in the emergency room. Slumping in the chair, I close my eyes. Rorschach blots of blackness drop beneath my lids as I feel a light sweat break out all over my body. Someone fans me with paper. "Put your head down for a moment, Mrs. Rawlins."

Yes. I know a cyclist.

Chapter 4

Doctor's Notes:

The patient had a Glasgow coma scale of six. His vital signs were otherwise stable and on a ventilator immediately on arrival at the emergency room. The patient's examination was significant for bilateral epistaxis. The midface was stable. The patient did have some road rash to the back. Trauma series x-rays were performed in addition to a head CT that showed a right frontal contusion, a left parietal epidural hematoma, a right nondisplaced skull fracture, a left mastoid fracture (near ear), a subarachnoid hemorrhage, a left parietal depressed skull fracture with pneumocephalus and a mild midline shift. The patient also had a T12 compression fracture, and a right orbital wall fracture. The patient was loaded with Dilantin and Mannitol and was emergently taken to the operating room with neurosurgery for evacuation of the epidural hematoma.

"Mrs. Rawlins," the chaplain prods. "You won't be alright alone. You need to call someone to be with you." She sits opposite me with Karen, whose nametag reads "Trauma Coordinator." *He'll be fine,* I tell myself. *In an hour, they'll come back and say the surgery went well and Hugh will be home in a few days. The doctor will have good news. Why are they trying to panic me like this?*

"Please call someone," Karen echoes softly.

"I could call my friend, Kelly, but she has small boys and her husband is away. I don't want to bother her."

Karen stares into my eyes. "Bother her! Call her now. You are going to need help!" Her firm tone shocks me into reality.

I fumble through my purse with a shaky hand to find a list of phone numbers. I can't remember any phone numbers. Hugh always remembers the numbers.

"Call your friend. It will be easier to wait with a friend. You also need to call family."

"They all live out of town. Should I really upset them like this?"

"Yes!" The word feels hurled like a stone. Softly she continues. "That's what family's for. They'll want to be with you."

A wave of nausea flips my stomach as someone grips my elbow and I'm shepherded to a seat placed directly beneath a wall phone out in the hall. Karen and the chaplain drift a few feet off, keeping me in sight as if allowing a child the breathing room to perform some newly learned skill under watchful eyes.

I call Hugh's mother, Rita, in Florida and tell her they need to come quickly, Hugh had a bad accident, he's having brain surgery. She cries, "No! No!" Between sobs, and with help from her husband, she says they will drive, so they have their car in Richmond.

Next, I call my own parents. I can barely control myself as I speak. "Oh dear God," my mother repeats. I want them to appear instantly. On a roll now, I call Kelly, my neighbor. Satisfied that I will have a friend, the chaplain holds my hand and offers a prayer before walking me to the surgical waiting area.

Kelly arrives by herself so quickly I wonder what she did with the kids. "The boys are fine," she assures me. Her blue eyes water over like shiny marbles. "I don't know what I can do for you, Rosemary. I don't even know what to say, but I'm here for you."

"Having you here is enough, Kelly. Thanks for coming. I don't want to wait alone."

We sit mostly in silence. There is no chitchat, no reading of waiting room magazines. Every so often, we look at each other, smile weakly, and look away. It's too painful to read each other's thoughts.

My friend, Debbie, Amanda's mother, arrives with her husband, Jeff. "The girls are at Skate Nation till ten," I say.

"I know, Amanda's with them," Debbie says.

"Would you mind picking them up from the party later and just tell them I'll be home soon? I want to talk to the surgeon before seeing them."

"Sure, Rosemary, I'll bring them over to my house. Don't worry about how long it takes." She engulfs me in one of her warm hugs. Jeff sits nearby, shifting uncomfortably in his chair the way men do when they can't fix something.

"I think I forgot to bring money for parking," I say. "I didn't know you had to pay for parking here."

Jeff perks up. "Here, Rosemary, take this." He pulls out his wallet and hands me five twenty-dollar bills.

"Jeff, parking costs $2.00 or something."

"Don't worry, just take it. You don't want to have to go to the bank. You might need it." His face is so sincere, and his gesture so kind, I stuff the wadded money in my pocket while thinking of all the days of parking this $100 will cover. Will I need fifty days of parking? The thought blocks my breath, like the shock of cold water after a high dive. My eyes squint as if trying make out images through a fog of smoke. Wedged into a corner of my chair, I feel oddly detached from everything and everyone. I'm told my husband might die today. Inside I chant, "Don't die, Hugh. Hold on."

Hugh's cycling buddies, Kevin and Rick, arrive and speak to the police officer who has just entered. They want facts.

"This could *not* have been Hugh's fault," Kevin says to her. "Hugh has been riding his bike for years and is a fanatic about safety. I know he was in the right lane and did nothing wrong. I would bet my life on it."

Ironically, Anna and Mary are the bike safety poster children for the school system. A picture of them riding along the road single file in helmets is portrayed on posters all over the county.

"We're still gathering information for the investigation phase," the officer explains. "The person that hit your husband is an older woman. As soon as I know more I'll get back to you." As the officer starts to leave, Kevin gestures her to one side and they talk quietly. I sit down trying to erase the pictures in my mind. Now I picture a distraught old lady having nightmares about the moment of impact.

At ten-thirty p.m., the doctor calls on the surgical waiting room phone to say Hugh is out of surgery and is resting in the Neurosurgical Intensive Care Unit, called the NSICU for short. It will be at least an hour before I can see him. Our minister, Keith Emerson, waits calmly with us.

"Where are Mary and Anna?" he asks.

"At their own birthday party. No, by now they're at Amanda's house. Debbie picked them up. I don't know what to tell them. I don't want them to see their father like this."

"Rosemary, they're old enough. I suggest you go through this as a family. Otherwise they'll feel left out and resentful. If you want, I'll go pick them up so you can stay here." I know he's right. I just cannot bear to feel the pain of all three of us together.

"No Keith, if you show up, they'll really worry. They'll think the worst." I take a deep breath. "I'll go," I say, "I can't see Hugh right now anyway." Kelly offers to drive me. Trying not to crumble, I greet the girls on Debbie's front porch and walk with them to the car. They exchange quizzical glances, wondering why Kelly is chauffeuring. Kelly offers them both a warm greeting while clearing the back seat for them.

"Mom, what happened?" the girls ask in unison as they step into the car.

"Dad's been in a bad accident. A car hit him on his bike."

"How bad is it?" Their hesitant voices pierce my heart.

"The doctors don't know yet, but he had an operation on his brain. It's pretty serious. Dad is strong, though. He's sleeping now. We'll just have to wait."

Back at the hospital, our friends and minister keep vigil. Word of the accident has spread. There are two waiting rooms, one outside in the hallway, and the other one right inside the NSICU for close family members. A nurse guides us into this small waiting area. Mary, Anna, Kelly, Keith, Kevin, and Rick arrange themselves around the circular table and I pull up a leather chair.

Once we're settled, the nurse speaks. "As you've heard, he came through the surgery and is stable," she says. "I just want to prepare you for what he will look like. He will have a lot of IVs and a bandage on his head from the surgery. He has a feeding tube and catheter. He has a brain injury that we are monitoring very closely and he may not be responsive. We will try to wake him up every two hours or so for neuro exams." Everyone listens intently. No one knows what a neuro exam is, but we don't ask.

Looking directly at Anna and Mary, the nurse continues with a firm tone, "Your dad is a very strong man in good physical shape. These things are on his side."

I notice the concentration on Anna's face. She often watches documentaries of real life surgeries on television. She wants to know all the details of Hugh's medical care. Mary is more sensitive, hesitant about seeing her dad in a hospital bed. She inherits her uneasiness from me. I always hated needles as a kid. My brother, John, loved biology. He often succeeded in grossing me out with talk of blood and guts.

I decide to go in alone first, to gauge my own reaction so I don't alarm the girls. As I walk through the ICU past several critically ill patients, I want to turn around and bolt out of the hospital. Then I see Hugh.

He is asleep. His face is perfectly unmarked beneath the bandage wound tightly around his head. I stare at his beautiful sleeping face before taking in his whole form. He's covered in sheets, hooked up to monitors and tubes. I approach cautiously.

"Hey hon. Can you hear me? It's Rosie. The girls and I are here with you. You had an operation but you're going to pull through this. I love you. Can you hear me?" No response. A chill of dread runs through me as I return to the conference room to gather the girls. When I enter, Mary is curled up in a straight back chair crying. Anna is stoic and quiet.

"Girls, Dad is sleeping. He looks okay. Want to see him?"

"I want to see him…but…I don't know." Mary's face is streaked with tears.

"I'll go," Anna says, as she stands up. I take her hand and bend toward Mary.

"Dad knows you're here with him, Mary. He knows you love him. He can feel it. I'm sure. You don't have to be standing right next to him."

"But I want to be right next to him. I just…" her voice breaks off.

"Take your time. There's no rush. You can see him when you're ready. I'll bring Anna. We won't be long." I squeeze her arm and her chin touches her knees as she sniffs and wraps her arms around her bent legs. Kelly draws closer to her and nods at me.

Anna strides boldly through the ICU, her dancer's back as straight as a stick. She stares directly at the other patients unflinchingly. When she first spots Hugh, she walks right up to the head of his bed, grips the railing, and begins speaking. "Hi Dad, it's Anna."

A nurse stands at the foot of his bed monitoring his vital signs. "You can hold your dad's hand and get close if you like," she says. Without hesitating, Anna takes Hugh's swollen hand in her delicate one and leans in to speak to him.

"Hi Dad, it's Anna. You look good, Daddy. Keep fighting. We're all here with you." When he doesn't respond, she shoots me a look of disbelief. "Daddy, I love you," she says in a shakier voice. When she hears no response, she glances at the bleeping monitor by his bed.

"What is that number in the upper right hand corner mean?" she asks the nurse.

"You can call me Kathy," says the nurse smiling. Here we have his heart rate—it's steady. And this one is his oxygen level. Ninety-eight is a good number." Anna stares at the machine. "Anna, I want you to know, I will be with your dad as long as he's on this floor for every one of my night shifts, and I will take extra special care of him. Okay?"

Anna nods, satisfied. She kisses Hugh's cheek. "Let's go back, Mom." We cling to each other all the way to the waiting room. A different nurse is speaking to Mary when we arrive. "I think you'll feel better if you see your dad," she's saying.

"I can't." Mary's eyes well up. "I just don't...."

The nurse repeats in a soft voice, "He looks different because he's been injured, but he's still your dad—nothing to be afraid of."

Mary looks at Kelly. "I will if you will," she says, and then she looks at me. "Mom, I don't want you to feel bad, but can you wait here? I'd rather go with Kelly."

My feelings are hurt. I want to be the one to comfort her, but I realize I'm a mess with red swollen eyes from exhaustion, not exactly the rock of Gibraltar right now. "Sure, Mary, whatever you want," I murmur.

Mary grips Kelly's hand as they leave the room. A thousand thoughts flood my head about Hugh, about Mary and Anna. How can

I help them? Coffee appears in front of me. I touch the cup but don't drink it. Keith is speaking, but I can't concentrate enough to hear him. Soon, Kelly and Mary are back. Mary appears a little calmer, relieved to have it over.

Now that the girls are settled, I return to Hugh's bedside. Kathy slips a chair beside me. "I doubt he'll wake up anytime soon," she says after awhile. "It's after midnight. He's in for a long hospital stay. You better go home and get some rest, even if it's only a few hours. You can call us anytime for an update."

I tuck the ICU phone number in my wallet, not wanting to go, but I know the girls will not leave me here alone—and I have the horrifying thought that I should tend to the living, our children. Before we leave, Keith prays with us. After a respectful silence, Kelly turns and says, "Rosemary, girls, can't I drive you home? You can get the car tomorrow."

Rick and Kevin walk with us to the parking deck keeping watch over Mary and Anna like surrogate fathers, the brothers Hugh never had. Kelly drives us home in silence.

Chapter 5

On the way home, scenes from our life together wash over me in a montage of split second images painting a wide streak of lush remembrance. In sharp focus, I see Hugh on the day we met at age twenty during a beach trip in the Hamptons on Long Island. A lean, muscular surfer boy with rugged good looks and chiseled cheekbones, he stands apart from the crowd and looks at no one. I cannot take my eyes off him. At six feet tall with rakish brown hair and a deep tan, he wears a tight shirt over hip-hugging powder blue bell-bottoms. He is the most handsome man I have ever seen. I intentionally bump into him.

I see him lying on the cheap webbed lounge chair by the pool in back of the motel where I stayed that night, his hands clasped behind his head, looking up at the stars. I fall in love with his beautiful face and quiet, unassuming manner.

I remember dinner in a wooden booth at Shippy's restaurant, sun-drenched beach days with Hugh's surfing buddies, walking in the sand holding hands while the wind blows salted hair strands across our faces, slow dancing at the OBI South. Days that turn to evenings that turn to nights we never want to end. We keep kissing through the screen door long after saying goodbye.

I see him standing opposite me at the altar in a white tuxedo on the day we marry, staring into my eyes calmly while I shake with laughter and nervousness.

I see him in our camping tent that springs a leak during a teeming rain; he's leaning on one elbow looking at me as if the sun is still shining. He laughs as I plunge in a fork and pull out a pot-shaped lump of glued together macaroni that I cooked on a hibachi fire in the woods. He's paddling a canoe down the rapids of the Delaware Water Gap after I lose my oar in an unexpected lurch of the boat, the ripples of his back straining against the pull of rushing water. We're playing cards in Chester Judson's cabin in the woods, he rubs his chin when he knows he's been dealt a bad hand. Later we make love on the straw mattress in that cabin, the old floor creaking in the stony silence of the forested night.

I see him in the kitchen of the first beach cottage we rented in Lindenhurst, Long Island, bare-chested in surfing trunks, ducking the raw hamburger meat I've just thrown at him in a fit of anger because he laughed at my inept cooking skills. He's charming our Italian landlady by sharing his pastry with her. In boxer shorts, he's bailing out the cellar flood after a rainstorm.

I see him running to catch his train to the diamond district in New York City for work and see him coming home late at night, struggling with career choices, changing jobs.

I hear him say, "Let's go off and make a new start. You always loved Vermont." Vermont—my grandfather's house on Crow Hill Road—the theater of my childhood vacations. It crystallizes in me like rows of spiky icicles that shimmer in the frigid afternoon light. I hear the crunch of his boots on hard packed snow; watch him savor the smell of crisp, clean air filtered by dense canopies of leaves. I see Hugh shoveling snow so high it builds a wall along the driveway. I see him graduating from St. Michael's College, smiling for pictures in his lopsided cap and gown. He's raking endless piles of orange and yellow leaves at our first house with the red front door and the chipped cement stoop. We're holding hands at the Church Street Marketplace in Burlington and feel like we're strolling along the inside of a postcard where fall foliage flutters down on us like confetti along the brick road, the old church with the rising steeple at the end. We sip drinks at Leunig's or

Sweetwater's, press shoulders in the dark Flynn Theater, and rest on the cool stone wall outside the Fletcher Free Library.

I delight in the surprised look on his face when I tell him I am having our first baby. I see his mouth round in disbelief and amazement when he learns we are having *two* babies! The morning his twins arrive, he says, "Most babies are so ugly, but these two are *so* beautiful and it's not just because they're mine." I picture him lying on the couch with Anna and Mary, two tiny living dolls sleeping on his chest, their heads almost touching at his collar bone, tiny bunches of his chest hair gripped in their dimpled hands. Hugh, with an infant in each arm at their baptism, long white gowns sweeping the floor. Hugh strapping them up carefully in their infant car seats and making faces at them in the rear view mirror.

I'm cheering Hugh on at the Howard Bank Bike Criterion with a twin umbrella stroller in tow. I jump with excitement when he passes his CPA exam despite zero sleep and midnight feedings. I see his broken front tooth after a Triathlon. He's pulling the girls in their red wagon in the fall and snapping their snowsuits in winter. I feel him next to me on the ski lift at Smuggler's Notch; see his Navy Thinsulate mitten resting on my thigh. Hugh at Terry and Tom's house down the street, in the garage they are always cleaning out. Hugh saying, "Terry, you know I hate peas!" and Terry always serving them anyway.

I see snapshots of Hugh waking up in the middle of the night to chase a nightmare away and rub a tiny back. I remember his perfect ears, small and pressed to his head, a sculpted, matched pair; the way his eyes change from blue to green to amber all in the same day; the way he surprises me with chocolate bars, the ultimate symbol of love for us; the way he touches me so gently it almost hurts for the intense desire it evokes.

I picture him packing up his car to drive to Richmond and start a new job, the long goodbye, the slow motion of unwanted departure. I see him in the pool at the rented Wellesley condominium, Mary and Anna splashing him, their chubby legs dangling and kicking water over the coping. We check on our new house taking shape in Glen Allen with a walk through the skeletal wood frame every evening, our toddlers scooped up to avoid landmines of staples, nails and splinters.

I hear the thunderous music while watching the fireworks after the Richmond Braves Game on the fourth of July at the Diamond; see the girls huddled against their father's brick hard legs, Anna holding her ears against the piercing pops and explosions. I see Hugh diving into the pool at the Hungary Creek swim club, slicing through the water with fluid grace and steady rhythm. I see him eating frozen Milky Ways under the umbrella at the round wooden picnic table. At the ocean in Florida, he's building sand castles with his cousin, Betty, and jumping over the waves with a gaggle of screaming girls.

A slideshow of Hugh with his girls runs through my mind: toweling slippery bodies after a foaming bubble bath, tying tiny sneakers, stealing their chocolate Teddy Grahams, watching them with rapt attention at their dance recitals, reflecting as they blow out the birthday candles year after year. I stifle a laugh at the thought of him squished on the sofa with them as he tries to stay awake through long Disney movies. His face goes soft on his fortieth birthday as he watches his eight-year-old girls sing "My Dad" to the tune of *My Girl*, while dancing with top hats tilted on their heads. His cycling friends surround them with sweat from beer cans dripping down their forearms. I envision him running beside Anna's mountain bike in the apple orchard beaming because she is the only girl in the race and she's beating the boys! I watch him listening to Mary tell him all about her day so earnestly. Her story winds around and around, but he never looks away; she holds his full attention and that pleases her. She tells him she'll only marry a man who shaves his legs like daddy. He does it to avoid ripping his hair with bandages after bike scrapes, but she likes the way it looks. Hairy legs are gross.

Then suddenly he looks like an executive in a business suit and tie, with flecks of silver at his hairline. He's holding a briefcase. Driving in profile with the car windows always down, wearing black Oakley sunglasses. Mr. GQ. He glows in candlelight at dinner out with friends. He stands by Patty King's huge wooden breakfast bar holding a napkin and eating a piece of shrimp, the room so crowded everyone's shoulders touch.

I see him straddled over his bike joking with Kevin, Rick, and Jim in the cul-de-sac before a weekend ride. Popping over logs on his mountain bike. Hanging out with Fred at Rowlett's bike shop.

He's embarrassed and tipsy after a few stiff drinks as he's pulled to the dance floor to learn the electric slide with all the women in his department at the company Christmas party. I hear him say, "Hi Hon" in the way he has greeted me at the end of every day for twenty-four years. I hear his exact tone and inflection and see him come into view, anxious for my response, eager to see me.

I hear the door close as he leaves for the office in the morning. Sometimes he leaves too early to say goodbye. I hear him on the phone, "Working late again. You know how it is." I sense him sometimes wanting more than I can give, wanting more from his career. I see him yearning, feeling the pressure of work, the monotony of long marriage, the pull of responsibility. Time has worn a path between us. We drift in the midlife doldrums unsure about our choices, wondering if we are growing apart.

All that changed today.

I see you, Hugh. I'm with you.

Chapter 6

Rosemary,

My thoughts and prayers are with you, Hugh and the family as everyone looks to the future and sees a remarkable recovery for Hugh. I believe this will happen and I know that as every second is filled with anxiety mixed with prayers, his body is healing. I believe he is in good hands and is being monitored carefully. I am here to support you and the girls in any way that I can, and/or that you need. We are spiritually bound – all of us on this earth – and whether spoken out loud or said silently, our prayers and thoughts are for Hugh, you and your family.

Love you, dearest Rosemary

-Letter left on the front porch with food from Bambi Jones, friend

Like an alarm, the car pops over the bump in our driveway and jolts me awake. Kelly's face looks worn. "Will you be alright?" she asks. I answer her with a weak smile before she drives back home. As we enter the house, I instinctively know that the slam of the front door is the sound of a chapter closing in our lives.

The girls mope around the kitchen, checking the fridge but not eating anything. "We'll be up early, so better get some sleep," I say. We hold each other long and hard in a tight huddle. "C'mon, we'll feel better if we get some rest." Reluctantly, they trudge upstairs.

I can't stand to be in the bedroom. Unable to lie still, I get up and pace the floors as if Hugh might show up at any moment. Looking out the front window, I notice the porch light illuminating a word spelled out in all caps: "HUPRMAN," the vanity plate on his Ford Explorer, a gift from the girls for Father's Day a few years ago when he had back surgery. The surgeon joked that he had to use a razor sharp knife to saw through Hugh's super dense bones, so this became his new nickname. Hugh was mortified by it; he detests people who brag. Now I look at the word and foolishly wish he *could be* Superman. I wish he had pushed back that car with his superhuman power. My chest cracks from the longing and aching inside as I walk from room to room. Each time I enter the kitchen, I see his shadow leaving for the last time, and hear the tapping of his cycling shoes as they echo on the kitchen floor. Finally, I climb the stairs, fall into bed, and sleep.

Thin bars of sunshine highlight the wall. It's morning. Rolling over, I catch sight of the framed poem on Hugh's dresser that Mary wrote for him as a Christmas gift when she was ten.

Life is just one big bike ride
It comes along with bumps and bruises
And long breezy cruises
Sometimes you're swift
Or you need a lift
There are mountains to climb
And hills to glide down
And interesting corners to turn around
When you're on the road
Watch out for cars..."

I can't read on. "Watch out for cars," I say aloud as I step out of bed and check the phone; no doctors have called during the night. Lee Facetti knocks at the door as I'm finishing my coffee. He greets Anna and Mary with a smile that softens his Italian brown eyes. His perfectly combed thick black hair, khakis, and button down shirt lend him an air of professional calm that defies the nervousness he expresses to me about seeing Hugh so incapacitated. He drives us to MCV while I deliver an update. When I'm done, I attempt a positive voice, "No calls last night. No news is good news, right girls?" Anna and Mary sit quietly.

Sensing their apprehension, Lee continually glances up at the rear view mirror and directs light comments to them. He lets out a hearty laugh when they tell him about their recent school dance. Upon entering the cavernous lobby of MCV, he tells a raunchy hospital joke helping us release our tension. The joke is not nearly as funny as our overreaction to it.

Stepping into the elevator, we head to the fourth floor fading into silence, each of us alone in thought, anticipating. As the doors slide open, Lee says in his executive voice, "Hugh is a fighter. If anyone can get through this, he can." The girls drift closer to him as we approach the ICU. Once inside the conference room they wait at the round table while I take Lee to Hugh's bedside where he lies sleeping. "Hey Hugh, Lee here. How are ya doing buddy?" his voice cracks a bit. Lee scans the tiny ICU area, the tubes, and monitors. "Barbara sends her love," he adds. After a short visit he turns to me. "Your husband is one strong man. I don't know if I could live through this. I think I would cave. He would be proud of you and the girls," he says.

Afterward, Mary and Anna enter Hugh's curtained off space with the fluorescent light over his bed. Anna presses kisses on his hands and cheek; Mary is content to stand by his feet. Anna whispers secrets to his sleeping form while Mary places pictures next to his bed, just in case he wakes up. We strain for conversation in the silence, the hours passing slowly.

By late morning, Jim and Electra find us. Jim is tall and reed thin from cycling. He and Hugh have ridden together for years. He's clearly upset. "This is a cyclist's worst nightmare," he mutters. "Who the hell did this?"

"From what I hear it was a little old lady," I say.

He mutters a curse under his breath.

"How are you and the girls holding up?" Electra asks. She shakes her head in empathy, swaying the mass of black curls as she listens. Her dark eyes seek answers beyond my words, in my tight jaw, my rigid shoulders. She's an experienced masseuse who can pinpoint body tension.

During the day, Hugh regains consciousness for short periods. His eyes stare vacantly when the nurse holds his eyelids open. I ask about pain medication and I'm told he is on a milky white substance, an amnesiac; there is little pain management due to sedating effects. The doctors need to see if he can wake up and respond on his own. The thought of Hugh not on pain medication sickens me. What if he's in pain but can't open his eyes and yell? The nurses assure me he won't remember a thing. But how can anyone *not* remember this?

Anna stands nearby. In her monotone voice, she says, "Daddy is down to two cc's of Vecuronium now, Mom." Anna keeps track of all Hugh's meds. She points to the monitor, staring down his vital signs, as if she can use her strong will to keep them stable. "Heart rate looks good, Mom."

Neuro exams are performed every two hours to see how Hugh's brain is functioning. The first time I see one performed, I have to hold on to the bedrails to steady myself. A nurse thumps Hugh's chest and says forcefully, "Mr. Rawlins, can you hear me?" With her thumbs, she pulls his eyelids open. His eyes roll, stop, and focus on her for a split second. She repeats commands to see if he can hear and understand her. The moment he looks aware, she shouts in a hurried voice, "How many fingers do you see, Hugh? How many fingers am I holding up?" His eyes roll into focus momentarily before his lids descend again, the way a door closes on an unwelcome intruder. Again and again, she gently pounds his chest and repeats, "Can you hear me? Wiggle your thumb if you can hear me. Mr. Rawlins, you are in the hospital. Wiggle your thumb if you can hear me." No response. She makes notes on her chart. Fear heaves in my stomach.

Mary sits in a plastic chair by the bed with her head leaning on her father's frozen shoulder, looking away from him toward the wall. Anna is glued to the monitor. The nurse asks if we would all like to participate in the neuro exam. "Patients often respond to family voices much better than strange voices," she says.

Mary looks up startled and says, "I think I'll take a short walk. I'll come back and rub his feet in a little while." Hearing her, I picture Hugh and Mary on our green leather sofa at home, each lying with their heads on opposite armrests, pushing and pressing each other's arches and toes, Mary's ballet-battered feet bending in response to the relieving pressure.

Anna decides to participate in the exam; her small oval face is serious. Pounding on Hugh's chest to wake him up, the nurse loudly says, "Mr. Rawlins, your daughter, Anna, is here. She's holding your hand.

It's your daughter—if you can hear me, squeeze her hand." Hugh looks like a rubber image of himself.

Then Anna speaks, her voice childlike, "Daddy, it's me, Anna. Squeeze my hand. Please Daddy…." And he does, hard. Anna jumps, "Mom, Dad squeezed my hand!" Inhaling sharply, she releases his hand and steps back, her face flushed and radiant.

Taking hold of the same hand, I squeeze and say, "Hugh, it's Rosemary, can you hear me?" He squeezes me back. In an effort not to lose the momentum, the nurse asks, "Mr. Rawlins, can you wiggle your thumb?" He does. Then he sticks out his tongue at her command. Everyone is wildly elated, stroking his arms, encouraging him. Medical notes are scribbled on the chart. Anna runs to summon Mary and she rushes to his bedside. Hugh responds to every one of our voices in one way or another, and we all know he senses who we are. He's thinking and reasoning. It's like witnessing a miracle.

Short periods of this are enough to exhaust him, so the nurse suggests a rest period. We take a dinner break and return to the hospital to find pandemonium. The front lobby is crowded with friends and well-wishers. My friend, Patty King, pulls me aside. "Just visit Hugh and take care of the girls—let everything else go now, Rosemary. Call me if you need anything at all," she says as she hugs me.

Krista O'Connell has come from Williamsburg, where she has begun post-graduate work at William & Mary College. She's been like our adopted daughter for several years now, ever since she attended the University of Richmond far from her Florida home. She is the daughter of Hugh's cousin, Betty. Betty's been like a sister to Hugh. "Aunt Roe, I'm so sorry this happened. I can stay and help until your parents come," Krista says. "I'll hang out with the girls."

We leave the hospital around ten p.m. elated and hopeful. The surgery is over. Hugh has responded to us and appears to be out of the woods. After showers and a late night warmed-over dinner, the girls listen with rapt attention as Krista tells them about dorm life. Before bed, they both give me a long hug, their sweet-smelling shampooed heads just tall enough to rest on my shoulder. "G'night Mom," they say in unison.

I place both cell phones in rechargers on the kitchen counter.

Upstairs, I set my alarm, so I can call the doctor who told me to check in with him when he makes his rounds from seven to nine in the morning.

Even though I feel hopeful after the day's events, I'm still unable to sleep. I look at the empty pillow beside me and get up for a stretch. My neck aches. I try to read. After two in the morning I finally drift off into the deep sleep of utter exhaustion, and then suddenly spring awake at four a.m. feeling strange and restless, not knowing why. Finally, around five-thirty, I shower and trudge downstairs to make a pot of coffee and call the ICU nurse for an update. Before my foot reaches the last step, I see bright lights blinking in the shiny reflection of the coffee maker. On the kitchen desk, the message machine of the home phone flashes furiously. A sick feeling rises in my throat; I have missed several calls. I had not heard the ringing upstairs.

When I touch the *play* button, the voice of a senior resident fills the room. He's asking me to call the hospital as soon as possible to give permission for another surgery. "Your husband has a clot developing in his brain and we want to do emergency surgery. His neuro exams are going down. Please call us." I immediately call and find out that the surgery is already underway; they did not dare wait another minute. Hugh had a walnut-sized blood clot on his right temporal lobe.

Feeling negligent, my voice cracks as I apologize to the resident on the phone for not being available. Guilt crushes me. "We acted as quickly as possible," he assures me. "But this second surgery is much more serious than the first. Your husband was traumatized by the accident and further weakened by the first surgery. This latest operation is pushing him to the limit." Hearing me moan, he goes on. "It's anyone's guess how he'll respond." His tone is somber. I feel the floor give out beneath me. The elation of the night before is far behind.

Racing upstairs to the guest room in the back of the house, I find Krista sitting up in bed, her short blonde hair tousled. "Krista, the phone rang last night and I missed it. Hugh is in surgery again. I can't believe I missed the call." I'm wavering in the doorway, wanting to be instantly at the hospital.

"You have to sleep, Aunt Roe. You have to rest. He's in good hands," she assures me. Unconvinced, I say, "I'll get the girls up. Can you get ready fast? I'd like to get there soon. Let's go!"

"Aunt Roe, don't feel so bad. You're doing the best you can. I'm sure he'll be fine. He's got great doctors." She steps out of the bed as I wake the girls and tell them to hurry, then I'm at a loss for what to do next. Krista takes a quick shower. As she enters the hall wrapped in a towel, she sees me standing alone, looking dazed.

"Are you alright Aunt Roe?"

All at once I'm crying like a baby into the shoulder of my tiny twenty-one year old niece.

Chapter 7

Three Days Out

In the hospital lobby, we wait again with our minister and several friends including a pale, gaunt Jim. Dr. John Ward enters the surgical waiting area following the operation. I rise to meet him, dreading the talk to come. Jim follows. "Can I be your other set of ears?" he asks. I nod yes, relieved to have a friend nearby.

The tall doctor gestures me toward a chair with calm confidence written on his face. In a positive voice he begins, "The operation went well. Your husband's vital signs are stable." He pauses as I take in this initial good news, then his blue eyes soften as he continues. "I removed a portion of Hugh's skull to relieve the swelling on his brain—to give it more room. The bone is on ice in the freezer. It will be replaced in about three months when his brain swelling calms down. Don't be alarmed when the top right side of his head looks like it has caved in—it will look like a deep dent the size of half a grapefruit on the side of his head and forehead. I promise you he'll look like himself again after the bone is replaced." I sit straight, not knowing what questions to ask regarding this surreal news.

"We have induced a coma with medication, meaning that we want your husband in a deep sleep so that his body does not have to do anything at all but heal." I draw back at the word "coma." Dr. Ward places his hand on my forearm, and leans in toward me. "We have successfully removed the blood clot from his brain and he came through the surgery in pretty good shape. All we can do is wait. There are basically three scenarios: number one: he could wake up and begin to recover and get well. Number two: he could take us for a roller coaster ride, have ups and downs, but recover. Or number three: he could die."

He squeezes my forearm. Looking calmly into my devastated face he continues, "I feel strongly that the outcome will be number one or two. Your husband is a strong man in good shape, Mrs. Rawlins. I think he'll make it; but I can't make any promises. He's been through a lot." I stare at the doctor as I take it all in. It's like trying to swallow a watermelon whole.

After an awkward silence, I say, "Thank you for saving his life again. Thank you." Tears cut me off. Dr. Ward stands and gives me a warm hug. As he turns and leaves, my confidence and love for this man are firmly cemented.

Jim and I look at each other as we walk away from the surgeon, both thinking of scenario number three: he could die. Instinctively, I don't believe it. I will not believe it. In my mind, I see a strong, defiant man. Hugh has always pushed the limit. Jim, who rides bikes with Hugh nearly every weekend, says to me, "You know how obstinate he is. He's going to make it, Rosemary."

We walk back into the lobby and everyone looks at us expectantly for news. Jim fills them in, and they disperse to call others with an update. Secluded in the private courtyard with Mary and Anna, I answer their questions, all of which ask, "Will Dad be alright?"

"I don't know but I think so. The doctor says he's real strong," I say, gathering them into my arms. As we reenter the hospital, I feel a soft veil of love surround me—the physical presence of prayer, holding in my sanity.

Once Hugh is out of recovery, I sit by his bed. A collar immobilizes his neck. Tubes violate him everywhere: in his nose, arms, bladder, and even from the top of his head protruding out of his brain. He is being fed, monitored, and pumped with life-preserving breath by these tubes so that his body works at nothing but healing itself. Doctors and nurses drone in the background as he lies sleeping. I want him to open the eyes I've looked into for twenty-four years. I feel certain they could communicate to me since he can't speak.

I watch my husband rotate, eerie as a lifelike doll, comatose and tethered to a turning bed. His body lies as morbidly stiff as a mannequin's, segmented by upright padded boards as though he's being packed and shipped—even the cooling blanket inflated with cold water to keep his core body temperature low, looks like bubble wrap.

The rotating bed moves slowly but constantly, first tipping him all the way to one side, so his right arm is perpendicular to the floor, then back to a flat position, then tipping left, to keep his blood moving. His face is swollen to twice its normal size with eyes like slits cut into its doughy surface. His eyelashes are gone, buried under the water pockets of his lids. Only arms, hands and feet are visible. His left hand is bruised and swollen.

Staring at his image, I ask the nurse, "How is the rest of him?" She draws back the blanket and the crisp white hospital sheet, carefully maneuvering around tubes and IVs to reveal his body. I gently touch his arm, chest, and legs, seeking answers. Pressure cuffs constrict around his calves, sounding as if they are moaning for him. Gauze pads in patches shield a raw road rash that scoured the skin on his thighs, hips and buttocks. "Better cover him up again," she says softly to me. While the nurse places the cooling blanket over his body, tears pour down my cheeks. Hugh hates to be cold.

To help him feel warm, I talk about the beach. I hope he can hear me and feel my words. Saying them melts my own eerie chill. "We're at the beach today, Hugh. The sun is hot on your shoulders...." The nurse leaves us alone for a few minutes. I keep talking about the beach as I take in the sight of his whole body. The only recognizable part: his beautiful feet. They are perfect, polished to a sheen by Mary over the years.

I am so lonely and so filled by him at the same time. I can hardly stand to look at him in this state, and yet when I do, I am compelled to stare, to memorize every detail of his damaged form. I peek under bandages, tuck in blankets, and hover possessively.

How can this be? We had a life plan. How do you live minute to minute with no real promise of an end game? The doctor says there is no prognosis; it's anyone's guess how far he may come. No one can tell us how much he's lost. I'm beginning to wonder who exactly lies within the head that has been shattered by the impact of that car. What does the future hold for us? I need to know, and yet I have found a strength I never knew I had and a certain peace in the present that comes to me in waves, informing me silently that things will somehow work out.

Anna and Mary generously apply their touch and pour loving words over their father like a soothing balm. While they visit, Dr. Ward enters the ICU and directs me to his computer. He shows me pictures of Hugh's CAT scan. When Anna joins us, he looks at me as if to ask, "Is this too much for her?" My smile tells him, "She's fine," as I allow her to squish in beside me and look at the images on the screen. Seeing a folder on the table, I read the doctor's notes:

Right temporal intracerebral hematoma. The patient is a 40-year old man who presented two days ago with epidural hematoma who became progressively worse following his left craniotomy. A follow-up scan revealed a blossoming right temporal contusion. With rising ICP (intracranial pressure) *and CT scan findings, evacuation of the hematoma was planned. The bone flap was left off and sent to the freezer.*

Turning to Anna's solemn face, I point out, "Look, they thought Dad was forty. He's forty-six. He'd be happy about that." She giggles before getting up and going back to Hugh's bedside, her curiosity satisfied.

Before we head home for a break, I stroke Hugh's hand and whisper softly, "We are at the beach again, Hugh. I can hear the ocean and see the girls jumping over the waves. It's a little breezy, nice and warm. I love you so much. Can you feel the sunshine on your face? Can you feel how much I love you? Keep dreaming about the beach." I hope to myself he is there, warmed by the sun, as he lies beneath a blanket of ice in the ICU.

"Ready?" Krista asks when she sees me leave Hugh's bedside, the girls by her side. She drives us home for dinner. The radio plays as we slip into traffic on the Interstate, but I'm preoccupied. I'm thinking about Hugh's ICU nurse; she advised me to start keeping a journal because Hugh will want to know what happened later on and won't remember. She says it will help me clear my own head, deal with my emotions, and keep track of his progress. I mention this to Patty King when she calls my cell phone in the car, and she agrees. The thought that this will drag on, and that Hugh won't remember gnaws on my nerves. *Don't think about that now.*

A forest of grocery bags, gift baskets, and floral arrangements has sprung up on the porch leaving only a narrow path to the front door. One plant is from Ken, a friend of Hugh's. A card is attached that reads, "My wife is a personal injury lawyer. We're here if you need us."

I hear the phone ring as I turn the key in the lock. Hauling packages into the kitchen, I see the red light blink on the answering machine. "We're so sorry…we don't want to bother you, but when you get the chance, could you let us know…" Mary grabs a pad, writes down all the names and numbers—people from work, people from school, from dance, from out of town. Anna packs food in the refrigerator and pantry while Krista places flowers in each room. The doorbell rings and the procession begins.

Our neighbor, Scott, hands me a Pyrex dish of sausage, peppers, and onions. "This is so nice. It's my favorite," I say. The brawny man stands there sweetly. A sad smile creases his eyes.

"What can I say, Theresa loves to cook." Behind him stands my friend Celeste with a platter of turkey rollups. She hugs me tight and the girls run to her for a hug too. Paul, from church, leaves a hot casserole without our even seeing him. The Pegrams deliver a tray of Hawaiian chicken. A few moments later, neighbors stop by, Jennifer and Tim, Chris and Tom, bearing spaghetti sauce, cakes, cookies, and salads.

Between these short visits, I am jumpy and disorganized. Krista sets the table. I return a few phone calls, but soon I don't feel like talking to anyone. Sitting down at my office desk right inside the front door, I compose an email to my five brothers and sisters scattered in Rhode Island, Atlanta, Tucson, Los Angeles, and New York. I know they will all be worried and want to do something, so I ask them to forward our news to the cousins and write Hugh notes and emails that we can read to him while he's in a coma. This will give Anna and Mary a way to pass the time with Hugh while he's unresponsive, and hopefully, Hugh will absorb the sentiment on some level of consciousness.

Glancing up, I see the business phone on my desk flashing with messages. I let them blink. Krista suggests I leave medical updates on my home answering machine for people who call while we are at the hospital. I take her advice immediately.

Slumped on the couch after a mixed up meal that includes a little of everything, the girls bring up the topic of school while Krista cleans up dishes in the background. Her khakis and summer sweater set look too neat and pressed for the messy work she's performing.

The girls are beginning to stress about missing classes, especially since we heard today that Hugh's hospital stay might be quite long. They're enrolled in the International Baccalaureate program, and they're concerned about keeping up with classes and homework. Mary and Anna often speak at the same time. As their words pour out simultaneously, they glare at each other for interrupting.

"Mom, the teachers are not going to let us skip work. We are going to have to make it all up," Anna says.

"You don't understand, Mom, even missing one day is really hard. We'll never catch up," Mary chimes in, as she tucks her legs under her and hugs a throw pillow.

"Do you want to go to school?" I ask them.

"No, we want to be with Dad, but what about school?"

"Dad is our number one priority right now. You can stay out of school and visit him every day for as long as you want. I'll talk to your teachers and they will understand. In fact, I don't really care if they don't understand. The last thing you need right now is something else to worry about." The three of us sink into the couch. Their small-boned shoulders relax.

"Aunt Roe?" Krista is gathering her bags and getting ready to leave.

The girls and I hop off the couch and take turns hugging her. "Krista, I can't thank you enough for getting here so fast and helping us so much," I say.

"I wanted to. My mom wants you to stay in touch and keep us updated. Give my love to Uncle Hugh and to your parents and sister. Are you sure they'll be here soon?" she asks walking through the front door.

"Yes, Kate called and said they're only thirty minutes away," I assure her.

We watch her car leave the driveway for the trip back to William and Mary. I know my kids wish they could return to life as usual too, they'd even do extra homework, as long as their dad was home again.

Chapter 8

Hey Hugh –

I wish I could be there to tickle your toes in person. You are all we are thinking about. I love you so much, big brother. You are my big brother, you know. I have looked up to you and admired you ever since that day you took me out on the ocean and introduced me to surfing. You made me feel confident and capable and not embarrassed to try—even if I failed. It is a gift you have given me over and over through the years—a true reflection of your generous and sensitive soul. I love you for taking such good care of my sister and for being such a great dad to Mary and Anna. You are in my heart. Rest well.

Love, Peg

- My sister in California

Days 3-7

Pop steps out of Kate's van under early evening clouds on April 15th, catches sight of me at the front door, and stretches out his arms as I run to his protective embrace. There is none of his usual gregarious greeting until he catches sight of Anna and Mary running across the lawn. "Bon Jour! Comment allez-vous?" he bellows. "Which one of you takes French again?"

Anna leaps into his embrace and shouts, "Me Pop!" A family orchestrated series of hugs, shoulder squeezes, and suitcase exchanges plays out all the way up to the porch.

The drive from Hudson, New York to Long Island and then Virginia has been grueling for my younger sister, Kate. "Thank you for bringing Mom and Dad here," I say to her.

"We all wanted to get here even sooner. How's Hugh doing?" she asks, squeezing her arm around my waist while she walks. Her other hand lugs a heavy suitcase. I nod and squint at her to say, "I'll tell you later" and she accompanies the girls upstairs to place bags in various bedrooms. My parents enter the kitchen and sit around the table with me. Before my mother even asks how I am, the tears flow. The three of us sit in silence except for my sniffing. My muscles collapse with relief in their presence. Mom squeezes my hand before she jumps up. "Your father's starving, as usual," she says. She chooses a casserole from the fridge as the girls tumble back downstairs, and after a quick meal, Kate drives us all to the hospital.

In the harsh light of the ICU, they see Hugh for the first time. "Nothing could prepare me for this," my mother says. She approaches the bed and pauses. The color drains from her face as beads of perspiration soak her curled silver hair. A nurse quickly grabs a chair and my mother falls into it putting her face down toward her knees. The silver cross she wears swings forward on its fine link chain. "Oh my God, I'm sorry," she says.

Pop approaches the bed and murmurs, "His face is still so perfect." My father's arm instinctively draws me to him in support. I lean on the softness of a well-worn blue and red plaid shirt he's donned for over ten years.

Mom takes a few deep breaths as she steps tentatively toward the bed. She has brought a vial of holy water with her, a gift her Aunt Dot guarded all the way from Lourdes many years ago. She lifts it out of her purse to place some on Hugh's forehead, and gingerly, pours a little above his eyebrows. The water quickly drips back dangerously toward his bandage. Instinctively, I lurch forward. "Wipe it up! It may have germs," I warn, as I pat the water off him with a tissue.

"It's holy water, Rosemary!" my mother scolds. I can imagine her sending out her silent apology to God for me, but I feel only slightly ashamed. "Thanks Mom," I offer, in a low voice. Dad withdraws to the waiting room to sit with his granddaughters and our friends gathered there.

In registered nurse mode, Kate carefully examines medical records, asks for clinical updates, and checks Hugh's vital signs. At thirty-nine, she looks more like a college student than a mother of three. Kate is the youngest of my five siblings. I considered her my private baby doll when she was a newborn and I was eight years old. She confers with me as both a nurse and a sympathetic sister. "They're doing everything possible and he is stable," she assures me. "This is a great hospital, Roe. But I'd love to meet the doctor tomorrow if I could—to get some details."

I watch as Mary gravitates toward my sister who is right at home in the hospital. During these first few days, she has instinctively sought other adults for consolation, knowing intuitively that I am on some separate plane, completely lost. Anna is single-minded in her effort to feel a sense of control. She keeps a constant eye on me, gauging my reactions, almost expecting her other parent to give out at any moment. She watches carefully and takes everything in, but I know she is hurting. I have heard her muffled cries in bed at night when no one is looking.

Later on, Ed and Margaret Martin visit. We have known them only a short time. Ed is a Methodist minister and surfer, like Hugh. The two men instantly bonded while taking turns on Ed's skateboard one night in our old neighborhood. Ed pulls Mary, Anna, and me aside. "Let's join hands," he says in the family waiting room, his pastor's voice like velvet. He looks at each one of us individually and thoughtfully, "Now, what will you ask God for?"

Mary speaks first. "I want my dad to live."

Then Anna, "I want him to live too, to wake up."

Ed turns to me expectantly. I think for a moment, and then firmly say, "I want Hugh to be whole again. I want a full recovery."

The girls shoot me an incredulous look, as if I had just asked the impossible. Ed's concerned eyes soften. "That's a tall order, Rosemary. Are you sure?"

"Yes," I respond. "It's the only thing he would want."

We all squeeze hands as Ed begins to pray. "Then that's what we'll ask God to do, trusting His will to do the right thing." With head bowed, Ed creates a prayer asking God for Hugh's life, for his strength, for his wholeness and for God to grant us the strength to share in that gift as it shows itself moment to moment.

As we release hands, Ed nods and respectfully steps away. He walks to Hugh's bedside, firmly grasps Hugh's shoulder, and prays aloud for his recovery. All of Hugh's vital signs calm down at the sound of Ed's voice. His breathing evens out; his heartbeat slows. There is no doubt he knows that Ed is with him. And in that knowledge he feels the presence of a spirit so connected, so in tune with his own, that he safely drifts into a peaceful healing sleep.

We leave the hospital around ten p.m. The porch light on our house illuminates a small package leaning on the front door as we arrive home in the dark. Approaching it, I see a gift bag containing two beautiful wire-bound journals with angels and stars painted on the covers. A simple note from Patty King is attached: "Pour your heart out on these pages." I slip the caramel colored one with the baby angel faces that look like Anna and Mary right into my canvas hospital bag.

The girls are nestled on the couch with their grandparents watching television. Kate can see me in the rocker from the kitchen. "Hey Roe," she calls, "Why don't you try one of the sleeping pills Dr. Ward prescribed for you today and see if they help you get any rest. You look wiped out." She hands me a pill and a glass of water. I swallow it, expecting it to take a while to kick in. Surprisingly, it works within minutes.

"Is anyone else in the room seeing double?" I slur, holding onto the rocking chair arms.

My daughters laugh. Suddenly, I slump a bit and Anna runs across the room to me. "Mom, are you okay?" she asks.

"I'm fine. I'm going to bed," I announce, but as I stand up, my hip crashes into the wooden banister.

Anna laughs again and puts her arm around me. "I'll walk you up, Momma." She smiles back at my sister as she helps me up the stairs to bed where I fall onto the mattress like a drunk, feet up in the air. Before leaving, she climbs on top of me for a long hug—the way she did when she was a baby. "I love you, Momma. Sleep tight." I fall into a dreamless sleep.

Waking up to daylight, I'm confused at first, and then remember we have a houseful of people and a lot to do today. Hugh's parents will arrive and see him for the first time. It has taken them a few days to drive from Florida. Stepping from the bed, I fill my mind with details instead of thinking of the emotional meeting to come.

At breakfast, I offer a plan. "Let's break up into teams. Pop and I will go to the hospital. We'll check on Hugh, and speak to the Nurse Clinician in the ICU. I'm sure she'll talk to Rita and Hugh and explain things before they see him. Kate and Mary, can you go to Hugh's parents' house and clean up a bit—maybe put on some tea?"

"Sure. Mary, do you know how to get there?" Kate asks. Mary nods yes.

"They're supposed to arrive around lunchtime. Mom, would you and Anna mind putting a quick meal together on your way over?" She smiles and nods. "We'll all meet back at the Rawlins' house at twelve. Okay?" Everyone swings into action.

Shortly after noon, Rita and Hugh Sr. pull into their own driveway. Together we welcome them and unpack the trunk. Once freshened up, we sit down to beautifully set table of chicken salad, rolls, fruit, and cookies, while we try to ease them into the reality to come.

As Kate drives us to the hospital, I notice my mother-in-law taking mental notes on how to get there. She has an amazing mathematical mind and a well-developed sense of direction. Rita and Hugh are both surprised at the size of the hospital and the massive eight-floor parking deck. It's a long walk up to the building. Once we step into the ICU, I introduce Rita and Hugh to some of Hugh's nurses before they are escorted to visit their son.

A nurse shows them to Hugh's curtained area. I follow. Hugh's father slowly approaches the head of the bed and speaks to Hugh. He tells him he loves him. He cries quietly, the tears of a man who has seen everything in World War II, including a kamikaze attack on his own Navy ship, but would have given anything not to see his son like this. Hugh's mother stays near the foot of the bed. She can clearly see Hugh, but keeps her distance. After staring a few moments, she turns and walks briskly back to the conference room. We all sit with Keith around the dark wooden table for a prayer. Letting out a long exasperated sigh, Rita says in a shaky voice, "I promised myself I would not break down."

"I think breaking down is totally appropriate right now," I say.

As I leave the family waiting room, Peggy Thibodeau, owner of the studio where both girls dance, rushes toward me. "Rosemary, I came as soon as I heard. I cannot believe this. How are the girls?" Tall and statuesque, she envelops me in a hug.

"They're managing. They've been great. It's bad, Peg." My voice breaks up.

Peggy guides me around the corner protectively, away from everyone. "How are you? Are you okay? Rosemary, I'm worried...."

"I am trying so hard to be strong. They don't know what this has done to him. God, Peg. I love him. I want to keep thinking he'll be okay, but no one will tell me that. He could die." Peggy looks stunned. I stand in the stark hall crying. "I need to get it together. I don't want the girls to see me like this. They need to have hope." Peggy digs in her large knapsack and hands me a crumpled tissue. I lean against the cold hospital wall, feeling my hair slide on the smooth surface—every cell in me weeping. "I feel like a crazy person. One minute I'm sure he'll make it and the next I fall apart."

Peggy steadies me. "It's okay. I understand. I wish there was something I could say or do, but you will get through this. Those girls are strong too. What can I do? I'll tell the girls not to worry about dance, and when they want to return, I'll even drive them. I'll do whatever you need...what else?"

"I don't know. Just pray." Peg leans in and hugs me until I can stop the flood of tears. Stepping back, I look at her stricken face. "Could you check on them now, Peg? I'll be back in a minute."

"Sure. Take your time." Peggy turns the corner and joins Mary and Anna. I hear her reassuring them. I straighten up and wipe my face before turning the corner to join the family, my face a pale and sticky mask.

I can't imagine the pain Hugh's parents are feeling. Hugh is all they have, their only son, named after his father to carry on the family name. His dad chokes up in the hall as he watches his twin granddaughters ahead of him with their arms linked. "He has so much to live for," he says, his voice quivering.

Looking up at him, I respond, "He will live. I can feel it. We all have to trust that he will." Saying these words out loud makes me believe them too.

At night, Hugh's parents offer me a ride home. They are both quiet. "I want you to know that whatever happens, whatever shape he's in when all is said and done, I will always take care of him," I say. "I will take care of him for the rest of his life. I promise you that; and not out of pity, but because I love him."

My mother-in-law turns to face me in the back seat with eyes turned down at the corners, she nods her head and says, "We know you love him, dear." Looking directly into my eyes, she mouths the words *thank you*.

Now that family is here, I can focus solely on Hugh, and spend most of my time at the hospital. My parents take Mary and Anna for walks to the gift shop or out for a hotdog at Jonathan's cart on the sidewalk outside.

Kevin, a physical therapist and one of Hugh's best friends, helps me pass the time with Hugh in a meaningful way. He shows me how to move Hugh's fingers and joints so he will not lose mobility later on when he is awake and active. In his instructive manner, he says, "Hugh's shoulder will be the first to go. It's good if you can keep up a range of motion by lifting his arm above his head and stretching his deltoids, especially as soon as he wakes up." Once he shows me, I quietly bend and stretch Hugh's finger joints, elbows, shoulders, knees, toes, ankles, and arches whenever I'm with him. While slowly stretching his arms over his head, I envision him paddling out over the ocean waves or shooting a basketball again.

During one of these quiet sessions, the ICU nurse talks to me. "Have you thought about hiring a lawyer?" she asks. "This is going to be a long expensive hospital stay." The card on the plant delivered to the house flashes in my mind. Ken's wife is a personal injury lawyer.

"I don't know," I mumble. The thought gives me an instant headache. I don't want to think about jobs, money, or lawsuits. I only want to stand here until my husband opens his eyes.

At home after dinner, my mind turns to Hugh's personal belongings that were given to me in the emergency room the day of the accident. I have not been able to open the bag with his torn, bloody clothes. I had thrown it in his home office. "Kate, I hate to ask you this, but could you check this bag and see if his wedding ring is in it?" The bag stinks of old sweat and dried blood. Kate takes it into the bathroom and searches through it. His wedding band is not there, but she finds a claim form indicating that the ring had been cut off his hand at the scene. Hugh's father is downstairs helping to clear the dinner dishes. When I show him the form, he offers to have the ring repaired for me.

As the week passes, Pop is intent on helping Mary and Anna escape from the sorrow drenched seriousness of the situation, if only for minutes at a time. He plays casino and slapjack with the girls at our kitchen table and sings songs with them in unison as he scoops up their cards. When they are not playing games, he's clowning with them and teaching them to waltz on the kitchen floor in full music teacher mode.

One night, while resting in a chair by the kitchen table, Pop swipes his face with a handkerchief, and openly cries as I sweep by him like a lost girl sounding out my positive hopes for Hugh. Anna and Mary gaze at him, their faces shocked at his sudden tears. "It's okay to cry when you love someone so much," he sniffs, and they run into his arms to comfort him.

Seeing my mother on the couch in her soft flowered robe, fingers wrapped around a mug of coffee in the morning, fills me with security. As a small child, I recited her full name with fascination: Julia Margaret Mary Flaherty Healey—the longest name in the world. Reflecting on her name I ask, "Didn't Pop's father used to call you 'My Jewel'?"

"Yes," she says smiling. "He was such a sentimental man."

"Mom, I hope I can handle this," I say to her. She covers my hand with her own. "I have no doubt you can handle it, Rosemary. You just have to go day by day. It's not going to be easy, though. Dad and I are here if you need us."

Kate's layered short blonde hair flops in her face as she kneels by the refrigerator and sorts through the contents to make room for the gifts of food lined along the counter. All of us Healey kids inherited Pop's work ethic. Actually, if we didn't inherit it, he ground it into us with this frequent reminder: "If you can't do something joyfully, then don't do it at all!" He actually lived these words. He worked long and hard to do his best, always with a smile on his face and a song that matched the task.

Toward the end of the week, everyone stays at the house one night while Jim drives me to the hospital. Seeing Hugh on the turning bed is unsettling. Jim, an avid photographer asks, "Do you think we should take a picture of him?"

"I don't know, Jim. It seems odd. I'm not sure I want to remember this." After a while we decide against it; there is a deep sacredness to Hugh's sleep that should not be invaded. There is also my unspoken fear of this being my final image of him. I have other pictures of my husband I want to remember for all time. Before we leave Hugh's side that night, I hang a prayer over his bed that Terry sent from Vermont:

God has huge hands, enveloping all of us. He holds the hands of the doctors, the nurses and all of us. But most importantly, he holds Hugh. My vision of recovery is a circle of love that is more intense than ever. We have, before, likened it to a bicycle wheel. Many spokes leading to the hub. Hugh is the center now and we are all his strength and his energy.

My family's visit comes to a close. On their last day in Richmond, we spend all morning and early afternoon in the hospital, before coming home to square a few things away. The dark sky and driving rain add to the dreariness of our mood. I need to find my Power of Attorney to get into one of Hugh's bank accounts, because the bank needs *his* signature. Never mind that it's physically impossible for him to sign papers. They insist on *his* signature. After a tense encounter at the bank with my sister where she watches me tearfully relay my story and spread the contents of my wallet on the counter—photo IDs, credit cards—I am still denied access to his account. A frantic search ensues back home. I don't remember where I filed that document. My father asks, "Don't you have a Safe Deposit Box?"

"Yes! That's it!" He is appalled when I pull out a Nike shoebox from under the bed with bright letters sprawled across the top in red magic marker: "Safe Deposit Box." It is a perfect visual for how unprepared I am for an emergency. At least the Power of Attorney is intact.

In her pastoral way, with a desire to soothe my sheared nerves, Kate lays out the blanket Mary and Anna are crocheting for their father. "The girls picked out the yarn," she tells me. "They decided that each color would have a meaning. Dark blue is for love, light blue for health, green for wealth and white for protection." In between visits to Hugh's bedside, she taught Anna and Mary to crochet in the hospital waiting room. The activity is a comfort to them and the blanket will provide a treasured possession for Hugh when he wakes up.

My parents and Kate pull out of our cul-de-sac on Friday, April 19th early in the morning. They all look as though they spent the night wide-eyed, staring at the ceiling. After waving goodbye, I find a letter on my desk in my mother's perfect penmanship with a check to buy Hugh a recliner when he arrives home from the hospital so he won't have to climb the stairs for a comfortable place to sleep.

I have long known and witnessed how much my parents give of themselves to others. Both have been my role models for many years. In my mind, there are two kinds of "helpful" people in the world: those who ask if you need help and those who help without asking. Mom and Dad are the latter – silent workers, like the wind at your back when you are running (or cycling)…so subtle you may not know the breeze is there, even when it's carrying you.

Chapter 9

Hi Uncle Hugh! Gee your name is easy to spell on the computer! The letters are all just right there! Anyway, I really hope you get better. I think about you every day! I heard that everything was doing good, and that really relieved me, because I got really stressed out on Monday. I hope you get better really soon. I love you soooo much! Bye for now. I'll try to write another note to you soon.
Love, Emma Waters
(You see, my name is hard to type on the computer, all of the letters are spread out!)

-Our niece, Emma, age 13, Tucson, Arizona

Days 7-8

Incredibly, my friend, Terry, had purchased tickets to visit us with her daughter, Rachel, months ago. Her flight is scheduled to arrive on the same day my parents and Kate leave. Only twice in my life has a close relative been taken to the ICU in a critical state. Both times, Terry had tickets in advance to visit me. This coincidence is just another one in a long series of parallels our lives have shared since the day we met while ambling around the block pregnant in Vermont fourteen years ago. Terry gave birth to Rachel two months after I had my twins. Hugh's parents offer to pick Terry and Rachel up from the airport and bring them to MCV later in the day.

In the morning, an ICU nurse talks to the girls and me while another nurse clears Hugh's lines. She keeps her back to Hugh's bed blocking Mary and Anna's view of the nurse bent over their father. He is still in a coma. "When Hugh wakes up, his personality might be changed," she warns. "He may be loud and angry or highly emotional and say inappropriate things. Some patients make funny noises and act in a way that is out of character. This is a frequent consequence of frontal lobe contusion called disinhibition, which is common in TBI cases."

Our faces seek each other out as she continues, checking each other's reactions. "People with disinhibition cannot control impulsive behavior. In other words," she says, looking directly at the girls, "if your dad says harsh or obscene things, it's because he can't help it, and he doesn't mean it, so don't feel bad." She notices that our expressions are morphing from tranquil to horrified and softens her tone of voice, "He may curse you out or call you names, or he might say sexually explicit things. Then again, he may not. We don't know yet; but we want you to be aware that it's just something that happens sometimes, and it may only be temporary."

The girls' eyes dart around the room like wavering turboprops seeking a safe place to land. Their pale and speechless faces settle on me. "It's okay, we'll be fine," I say to the nurse, "Like you said, it may not happen." I hope they can't see my heart beating wildly through my thin cotton shirt. I'm relieved to see their faces visibly relax.

"Okay," says the other nurse, "I'm done here. You can visit your dad now." She smiles an efficient smile as she coils a long rope of plastic tubing. Placing a few cards on the bed stand, the girls talk quietly to their father and read to him from the notes and emails he's received.

After a little while, they ask if they can go to the waiting room to do homework. Diana Stone, a church friend whose son attends the same middle school as the girls, had visited earlier in the week, nudged them affectionately, and said, "Hey girls! Don't think that just because you're here you won't have any schoolwork. I'll pick it up for you and deliver it." She has been good to her word, bringing stacks of homework daily.

"Stop back up here when you're ready to go to say good-bye to Dad," I say, and off they go.

A tall female physical therapist pops in, introduces herself to me, and studies Hugh's chart. "Mis-ter Rawlins," she says to herself as her eyes scan his history. I watch her deftly reposition his sheets, grip the heel of his foot, and apply pressure. After concentrating a second, she cheerfully announces, "He's pushing back."

The nurse, flicking his new IV bag, turns around and says, "I don't think so," in a flat voice.

The PT pushes his foot harder. "He is. Feel this," she says. The nurse reaches for his foot and presses her hand palm to heel. Sure enough she feels a slight pressure in return. With a curl of her finger she motions me over. I mimic their exam but don't feel him moving. "It's a slight pressure," the PT says, "but it's there." My heart skips with joy when I think I feel something, then thuds when the nurse says, "He's coming around, but it takes time. It may take hours for him to open his eyes. We're slowly reducing his drugs." I think to myself that waking up from a coma is nothing like the soap opera version.

The PT makes her rounds and returns again to check on Hugh at intervals. Each time he moves a bit more, but barely. My head throbs with anxiousness. Finally, near noon, he opens both eyes in a startled unblinking stare, a lifeless gaze. The absence of his soul—his blankness—hits me like a jab in the chest.

Hugh responds to voices, but only by moving, not speaking. It's hard to tell if he registers anything more than discomfort. I sink back in my plastic chair. What has all this done to him—to the person that is my husband? My fantasy is smashed—the thirty-second triumphant scene where Hugh's head turns on the pillow toward my voice, his eyes open, clear and bright, and he says, "Honey, what happened?"—I have anticipated this magic moment hundreds of times during the past week. It's the Pisces in me, the dreamer, made stronger by the monolithic happy gene my father passed to me.

Any moment now, I keep thinking he'll come around, maybe even scream, ask me why he's in the hospital. Hugh's eyes flutter again making my expectations rise, but he quickly falls back into the cavernous black hole of unconsciousness. I let out an exasperated sigh. The nurse explains that waking up often takes time. He will gradually gain his bearings and will slide in and out of wakefulness. While I wait in this pressure cooker of anticipation, I hear a familiar voice.

"Rosemary!" It's Terry. I'm enveloped in a hug. Opening my eyes, I see Rachel beside her. Terry looks down at Hugh on the bed and says,

"God, I feel so helpless. I don't know what to say." Helplessness is the feeling Terry hates most in the world. She is a friend who wants to fix and heal. As a former EMT, she comes by it naturally. Her tall frame leans over Hugh's bed inspecting the damage. She pushes a curl from her forehead; her thin high-arched eyebrows frame dark blue eyes that mist over at the slightest provocation. "This is *unbelievable*," she murmurs, "So this is what *critical* means. My God! It could easily be Tom in this bed."

Back in the lobby we find the girls. Rachel slams into Anna and Mary in a three- way collision hug. Her high volt energy is a welcome diversion. Rachel's reactions are heartfelt but short-lived. When she sees Hugh, she is devastated, but five minutes later, she has the girls involved in a whirlwind trip to the gift shop to find the funniest greeting card. Terry and I sit by Hugh, and I talk to the visitors that show up at the hospital, but there's little change. After evening visiting hours, the nurse suggests we head home. She assures me he will not be dancing the jig anytime soon.

In the van on the way home, Terry and I can hardly hear each other as the three girls chatter in the back seat catching up. One of them yells up to us, "Hey, tell us about the time you both got off the plane in Washington, and you were wearing the exact same new coat!"

Terry shouts back, "Yeah, it's weird, we did do that. A few times we bought the exact same thing in the same week several states apart without knowing it too: there was that silver teapot and the colorful welcome mat."

Once home, Terry mines through my pantry for ingredients to create a one of a kind meal while I sort through the pile of mail on the table, not intending to open any of it. Terry is a freestyle gourmet cook and lover of fresh foods. Settling on a spontaneous blend of pasta, olive oil, herbs and veggies that she finds in assorted gift baskets along the kitchen wall, she combines ingredients without fanfare or precision. Standing by the stove with a cold beer nearby, she pinches green flakes into the pan and says, "Measure to your taste buds!" We talk at length while she chops, tosses, and serves. I light a candle as we settle at the table for dinner, savoring the connectivity of lovingly prepared food and friendship. Terry takes a forkful of pasta and says, "Hey, I'm thinking I should take the girls out tomorrow so you can visit Hugh alone at the hospital. How does that sound?"

"Oh, Terry, that would be perfect. The girls could really use a lift and I want to talk to the doctor alone. I'm sure I can get a ride to the hospital from a friend if you want to use my van. Do you want some directions around town?"

"Nah, we'll figure it out. It will be an adventure. The girls can help me, and if we get lost, that will be fun too. We'll meet up with you at home later in the afternoon. Rae will be so happy to spend time with Anna and Mary."

This Saturday morning sounds just like the Saturday morning of Hugh's accident when the girls were getting ready for their skating party. Both showers run, footsteps thump above our heads in the upstairs rooms, and the girls are swapping clothes with Rachel for their day out. Downstairs, I phone Kevin's wife, Donnelle, to ask for a ride to the hospital. She appears in the driveway right after breakfast.

Sitting by Hugh's hospital bed, I'm anxious about his personality. This is a disorienting day for him as he emerges from the fog of drugs that induced his coma. Struggling to communicate, his voice is more like a crackling breath, low and scratchy, than a regular speaking voice. Leaning down to hear what he is saying, I feel sure it is something very profound.

"Ta. Glah. Ah." he says faintly.

"What are you saying? Try again," I urge, squeezing his hand.

He repeats the same phrase over and over, a short sentence I can't make out. Restless and uncomfortable, he croaks between bouts of agitation when he grabs at tubes and thrashes around the bed, one time spastically throwing his right leg over the side railing, which unnerves me so much, I fall back in my chair panting.

Pinpricks dig in my neck, creating a stiff ache from leaning over to listen, and my head throbs with frustration. I have waited seven days to hear him speak and now I have no idea what he is trying to tell me. By the end of the afternoon, the nurses and I finally make out what he is saying.

"Take my glasses off."

"What?" I ask, incredulous.

"Take my glasses off."

"You don't wear glasses, Hugh." He repeats the same sentence again and again. Finally, it occurs to me that he thinks the tape on the bridge of his nose is a pair of glasses because it itches. I scratch the top of his nose and he relaxes. Is he immersed in a dream world where he's wearing irritating glasses—maybe at work? Or is he just living in the moment, consumed by an itch and all the strange feelings in his body?

Now that he can move, he goes to the complete opposite end of the spectrum—from comatose to agitated—as he tries to pull out all his tubes and IVs. He's reacting to discomfort without understanding where he is or why he's there. He has to be restrained, tied to the bed for his own protection; otherwise the feeding tube will have to be reinserted constantly, a process that is uncomfortable for him and time consuming for the nurses. The restraints are necessary but seem cruel to me. Now he's tied down like Gulliver, arching and struggling against the ropes. I untie him every time I sit with him and keep his hands in mine. It's like trying to soothe an irrational giant. What's more, I'm not sure he knows me. There's no glimmer of recognition, only random thrashing about.

The doctors initially think that Hugh will need another several days on the breathing tube, but it's taken out at ten a.m. I'm told to expect the oxygen mask to be on for a few days more, but the respiratory therapist checks him and it comes off within two hours. His oxygen level is normal and steady. I remember how Hugh used to play with my peak flow meter, a gadget asthmatics use to check their exhalation force. I registered a 350. Hugh blew the top off the plastic tube at over 700 with his athletic lung capacity.

A food tube snakes through his nose to his stomach and delivers food and meds to his system. "Pull it out!" he keeps yelling to anyone nearby in his strange new raspy voice. One of his nurses tries a silk tube that is thinner and thought to be less irritating. "Take it out," he grouses. This stranger's voice coming from my husband's mouth makes me wince. He speaks only in short abrupt sentences devoid of emotion. I think that he's aware but unhappy when we are talking, but the doctors tell me not to be worried, he is not himself at all yet, and won't remember this.

"Calming Hugh is like wrestling an alligator," a muscle-bound male nurse says. "Your husband is one strong man, Rosemary." I hear that phrase over and over again. Later, when I'm standing up holding his hand, he suddenly pulls me closer. His grip is tight. With my elbow bent at a right angle, he yanks and I'm off my feet so quickly I nearly fall on top of him. Is he dreaming or intentionally pulling me? Suddenly my own husband scares me.

One minute he looks asleep, then suddenly his eyes fly open, they look aware for a few seconds, but not long enough that I feel like he knows me. I really want to talk to him, so when I have a private moment, instead of asking what the nurses ask, "Do you know where you are? What is your name? What year is it?" I get more personal.

Rubbing his forearm, I speak calmly, "Hi Hon. Do you remember your daughters?" His eyes are closed, but his lids flutter. I wait a few seconds.

"Mary...Anna," he croaks out slowly.

"What color hair does Anna have?"

Very softly he responds, "Yellow." I am smiling.

"What color is Mary's hair, Hugh?"

"Brown." I'm giddy. This begins to feel like some weird kind of date.

Then I ask him, "Do you know who I am?"

He responds, "Wife – Rosemary." He is speaking low, almost inaudibly; sometimes with eyes closed but now he opens them for a second. Our eyes lock. "How old am I?" He stares at me intently for a moment. I hold my breath.

"Beautiful," he replies. Then, his eyes close. He's instantly asleep. I relive that moment a thousand times and tuck it away as a memory to keep.

While he's cognizant only a few seconds at a time, I feel hopeful. He mostly grunts and complains about the tubes. I want to respect his dignity. I don't want other people to see him like this, but it will be difficult with so many genuinely concerned friends. The nurses advise me to be direct and firm, only allow a few people in, and keep visits short, but it feels as if there are so many people involved, so many that care.

How can I explain this to them?

Hugh is a private person who made it his rule not to discuss politics or money matters unless he is very close to someone. He conducts himself in a professional manner, unaffected by sentiment and convention. He always considers and analyzes before speaking or acting, keeping opinions and criticisms largely to himself. Would he want others to see him in this state? Buried beneath a mountain of confusion with waking moments that are unpredictable and bewildering, he sometimes blurts out inappropriate comments that I know are not part of his usual behavior. I wonder if he's said anything offensive to anyone when I'm not around, perhaps to someone that might not understand that his brain is misfiring. Limiting visits, especially from his co-workers, may afford him a measure of dignity at this stage of his injury.

I wonder if he thinks he's asleep. I've sometimes dangled between sleep and wakefulness, not sure which was which. I can only guess what he is feeling and how scared he might be when he senses reality surrounding him – the harsh lights, IV drips, and white coats, especially when I'm not with him.

I forgot to plan a ride home in the afternoon. Terry is still off with the girls. I drag along the hallway, emotionally wrung out. Hugh is fast asleep and will be knocked out for hours. As I walk out of the ICU, there stands my friend KiKi, as if summoned.

"Rosemary, I've been trying to find you. Is there anything I can do?"

Relieved, I hug her and say, "I need a ride home. You're just in time." In the car, we talk mostly about Hugh until we arrive at my house. KiKi pulls in front of the mailbox around four p.m., but won't let me leave until I promise to call her if I need help. I tap the car window affectionately as she pulls away. Not until I reach the top step of my porch do I realize that I'm locked out of the house. I don't have my car or house keys since Terry has them, so I lower myself onto the front steps outside, remove the sweater that I wear in the frigid ICU, and enjoy the late afternoon sun on my face. The accidental break is welcome—no bleeping machines or medical discussions.

Glancing out over the cul-de-sac, I see signs of spring emerging. Lawns are greening up, creating a vivid background canvas for colorful bunches of wintered-over pansies. The baby daffodils I planted last fall have already bloomed and droop lazily, their mini hats sweeping the dirt. Azaleas burst with color in a variety of pinks. Floating white dogwood petals hang in the distant back yards between houses. The neighborhood is under construction and not entirely finished, but our area is done for the time being, the last remnants of timber scraps and abandoned vinyl siding hauled away. Our little round of houses is populated mostly by young couples with small children. Heather, Madison, and McKenzie run from house to house across the way, busy in their childhood games, their motorized toy vehicles abandoned in the street. Several neighbors stop by to talk, and before long Terry pulls up with Anna, Mary and Rachel. For a short while, I forget that my husband lies critically injured in a hospital bed, until I feel a draft of guilt for severing my emotional tie to him even for a moment.

The house opens, dinner preparations ensue, and a fashion show fills the next hour. "Look, Mom, Terry bought me this. Isn't it cute?" The girls run excitedly up and down the stairs, grabbing dinner in snatches and talking about boys. After eating and picking up, we pile in the van and trek back to the hospital for a few hours. Everyone visits with Hugh and takes turns talking to friends in the outside waiting room. Terry coaxes Hugh, hoping for a response. "Hey, I brought you some peas!" she jokes while rubbing his arm, but he lies still as a statue. Her concerned face glances up at me with a deep sense of sorrow. "C'mon, let's go home. He's asleep for the night," she says.

I groan as I fumble with keys on the dark porch when we arrive home because I forgot to turn on the outside lights when we left. From the porch, the ringing phone sounds like a nagging screech. Inside, messages flash, and Terry's eyes scream, *this is insane!* The girls run upstairs. I answer the first few calls. When the phone rings again, I see Terry's face say *don't answer.* "It's my sister," I say. "I'll just be a minute." After hanging up, tears fill my eyes. "I don't even want to be here. I wish I could sleep at the hospital." Terry takes the phone from my hand.

"You can't," she says, "You have to take care of yourself and the kids." She pours us both a drink and hands me a glass of red wine. "Here." She nods her head as if to say, this *is good medicine."*

Seated in my office on a white striped sofa facing the computer screensaver of shooting stars, I scan the surface of my desk then look away, unable to consider all the papers, cards, and notes that need attention. Terry's knees are drawn up to her chest and she's facing me, her elbow bent on top of the couch pillow. It's our first real chance to discuss the day's developments privately.

"What are the doctors saying?" she asks.

"Nothing really, they just don't know. They say it takes a long time."

"But how long? Will he get better?"

"No one can tell me. All they say is to be patient. We have to take it day by day."

"Does he know what's going on?" Terry leans toward me, expecting answers.

"He doesn't appear to. He's really out of it. He doesn't know what happened or where he is." I stretch my neck from side to side to work out a kink. We hear it crackle.

"What about the future? Did they tell you how long it usually takes?"

"No one knows. Every case is different."

Terry falls back on the couch pillows; a look of exasperation sharpens every feature on her face. "*How* are you going to do this?" she cries in a desperate voice. Her big blue eyes spill tears as she sets her glass on the file cabinet and wipes her face with a loud sniff.

"I just am. I have to. I'll be okay." I bite the cuticle on my pointer finger and my eyes water up again. Silent, we curl into a seated fetal position, knee to knee staring at the unfinished work that litters my desk.

"You're not going to be okay. You're not! How can I help?" She looks at the phone flashing across from us, demanding attention.

"None of my clients know about Hugh's accident. People want job quotes and want to know if their résumés are done. I'm in the middle of a few jobs! My poor clients! I'll never get to it…they won't have…"

"*Your poor clients?* Are you kidding me? You can't work, Rosemary," Terry says firmly. "You have to shut down here. I'll help you put something on that machine. How about this!" She stands up and lifts the phone off the receiver, speaking into it as if recording a new 'away' message. In a strained, harsh voice she says, "Hello. I'm either at the ICU or away from my desk. Don't you dare leave a message because I can't do one more damn thing right now!" My eyes grow wider as she continues, "Or, how about saying, 'Hello. What the hell do you want? You think you have problems, well listen to this!' That will make them hang up!"

We fall over laughing on the couch, then I stand up and add, "How about this: I can't come to the phone right now because my husband's in a coma and I'm going *out* of my *fucking* mind but I hope YOU have a nice day!"

Terry bursts into laughter, then looks up in mock seriousness and says, "Hey, isn't it supposed to be Hugh that says inappropriate things? You're the one with the filthy mouth!"

"Oh shut the fuck up!" I say. She throws a pillow at me screaming with laughter. We're holding our stomachs in uncontrolled hilarity when we hear the girls scamper downstairs.

"We have a performance for you!" Clad in colorful costumes from the seventies, they line up like divas and sing at the top of their lungs, "She's a BRICK...HOUSE."

Terry and I yell back, "She's mighty mighty!" We throw up our hands, and bump hips. For a few minutes, we're transported to the fourteen-year-old world of the here and now. We want to be young again, able to step in and out of this crushing reality as seamlessly as they do. After the song, our smiles meet, and we break out in a round of thunderous applause, leaning in for a group hug. We all wind up in a puppy dog pile of exhausted silliness.

Later on, in the stillness of the night, after everyone is tucked away, I touch the empty pillow beside me again and smile inside because I heard Hugh speak today. He called me beautiful. I fall into a deep, vivid dream. I am running in silence, yet I know a small nation of onlookers is cheering for me and urging me to the finish line. My arms pump hard and fast. My heart beats strong. The sky, a blue wash, is painted over with watercolor clouds and the air smells sparkling clean. I feel like I can run forever and never tire. My lungs seem to take in gallons of air as I glide down the road in perfect stride, powerful and in control.

As dawn breaks, I stir with the half-light and try to drift back into my dream, but I'm awake and reality hits. "Let me be that strong, God, let me be that strong," I pray as I leave my bed to start another day.

Chapter 10

Sunday April 21st
Journal entry to Hugh

Today is Sunday. Yesterday I asked the nurse to put a cap on your head so the girls would not see the roadmap of staples and dried blood, and the drain tube coming out of your brain. It's pretty nasty. As usual, the girls were happy just to be with you. Today you are so tired but won't sleep. You are not complaining about the food tube. Your right hand is very active, squeezing, pulling on our rings, stroking our hair, and even pulling us into the bed. Your left side seems weak.

Days 8-11

The nurse explains, "Hugh's hand activity is called *picking*, a part of the agitation most brain injury patients experience when they first wake up. Many patients grab and pull at things constantly. A quiet environment with low stimulation usually helps. Lots of visitors, noise, and activity will contribute to increased agitation." To keep Hugh calm, we visit in small groups intermittently, and call it a night at eight-thirty.

Our kitchen at home has become a container for gift baskets. We have far more than we can eat, so Terry and the girls make a project out of sorting and stocking the pantry. We pack up one of the fruit baskets, add some smaller snacks, and deliver it to the ICU nursing station with a thank you note early Monday morning. Our visit is quiet and uneventful. Hugh is restless but not cognizant.

At noon, Terry and I walk with the girls to a peaceful lunch spot in full sun by a fountain on the corner of Twelfth and Main in Richmond. It is Terry and Rachel's last day with us. The girls balance on the brick wall that surrounds a fountain, while we listen to a street saxophone player perform a blues song on the sidewalk. Ambling back to the hospital, Terry puts her arm around my shoulder protectively. That afternoon, she makes a final effort to break through to Hugh. He does not recognize her. Outside of his room in the hospital hallway, she confides in me, "The worst moment of this whole trip is saying, 'Hi Hugh' and … nothing…nothing…nothing. God, Rosemary, I hope he's not dead to his old world!"

Emotionally exhausted, Terry loads the car with her suitcase just before dawn the next morning. "I tossed and turned all night. I can see why you never sleep," she says to me. While driving to the airport, I'm anxious to return to the hospital. At the curb, the girls hug Rachel and promise to write. While they chase each other playing Gotcha last, Terry grabs her luggage from the trunk. "You don't really need company right now," she says. Turning to face me, she continues, "It's so clear that this is just about the two of you. You need to be together to get through this—you need to be connected to him every second. It's so strange; I can almost see this force pulling you all the time. You better go. We can get to the gate from here." A tight embrace, and the girls and I are back on the road.

Turning onto the highway, I review the facts as they spill out of the hiding places tucked in the denial folder of my mind. My husband is not going to wake up and be the same old Hugh. Doctors and nurses have all been telling me it will be a long, slow recovery. I've heard the laundry list of cognitive impairments and neural complications that may affect his physical, intellectual, mental, and emotional well-being. It hasn't really registered yet. Maybe I'm stubborn and defiant, or maybe I am just plain unwilling to accept it. I picture injuries as physical bruises and broken bones. I have no experience that tells me how to deal with a brain injury, no idea what's ahead. I feel as prepared as an unsuspecting beachgoer before a tsunami.

Doctors and nurses slowly spoon-feed me the more frightening details of Hugh's long-term recovery. I find their passive delivery of his catastrophic condition mind-blowing.

"Will he be able to walk, drive, play sports? Will he ever work again?" I ask.

"We don't know. Time will tell," they reply.

"How much time will tell?" I ask.

"We really can't say at this point."

"His injury is serious, does that mean he won't heal as well?" I ask.

"It's a strange thing. Some heal fine, others don't. You just have to wait." Finally, I stop with the questions—they make me crazy—they bore holes in my sanity.

Hugh's coworkers are calling the house to schedule visits, but I put them off. I can't tell them, "Hey, this is what's wrong and this is how we're fixing it." I can't tell them much of anything.

Before April thirteenth our biggest problems were the daily annoyances of life—a long line at the grocery store, a slow-moving traffic jam. Now I have a thin booklet entitled *Rehabilitation and Research Center Brain Injury Manual,* that cites the possible challenges Hugh could face as he deals with this injury: seizures or post-traumatic epilepsy, hydrocephalus (fluid on the brain), insomnia, depression, hypoarousal, hypoattention, agitation, joint contractures, hypertonicity (muscle and arterial tension), clonus (involuntary muscular contractions) and spasticity, bladder incontinence, dysphagia (problems swallowing), deep venous thrombosis, breathing and movement problems, impairment in the special senses, and perceptual, communication or cognitive problems.

I find myself Googling medical journals and dictionaries late at night trying to decipher medical terminology for hints of what may come. I have read stories about people with brain injuries that make me fall back on my pillow and hyperventilate in fear when I learn about personality changes, violent tendencies, job losses, and depression. Where are the happy endings? Are there any?

With a mind full of medical jargon, I drive the girls back to MCV while I quietly resolve to find some answers. The girls are in the care of their sullen, preoccupied mother. I look through the windshield, driving mechanically, and wonder how this is affecting them. Will they wind up on the psychiatrist's couch in ten or twenty years because I handled this all wrong? I don't ask what they're thinking because I know they want answers, and I don't have any.

Hugh is tired when the physical therapist drops in and says she will try to get him up. His parents arrive and sit with us, exhausted from the long trip into the hospital. The strain is etched on their faces. As we visit in pairs so Hugh can have time with each of us, Hugh's mother speaks to me about his Explorer. "There are a lot of miles on that car, Roe. I know it's been acting up. Get it checked out and have the works done. I want you and the girls to be safe. Dad and I will pay for it." I still have my blue van to drive while the Explorer is in the shop, so I take her up on the offer.

Hugh's father pulls me aside later and hands me a tiny item wrapped in paper. Inside I find Hugh's repaired wedding band. I tilt it to read the inscription: *RH to HR 7-1-78 Forever Yours.* Hugh's father smiles down at me and I smile back, squeezing the ring. It feels solid in my hand. I slide it on my finger, but it's too large, so I add it to the chain around my neck for good luck, determined to place it back on Hugh's finger someday. I think about our wedding day in a way I haven't in years. The image of him young and strong, happy and committed to our future, makes me yearn to have him back the way he was. We will be married twenty-four years in July. Back then I never gave a thought about how long we'd stay together.

The blending of our lives was difficult at first; our families were so different. Whenever he was out of our apartment, I was lonely. But as an only child, he needed some time by himself. We had a stormy first year of marriage and several furious fights with passionate make up sessions.

When Hugh was growing up, his household was quiet and reserved. Neither parent liked television much—they were readers. Mealtime was civil and proper. I grew up with five brothers and sisters and a live-in grandmother whom I adored. We were a loud, dramatic family. Mealtimes were noisy and fun, all nine of us packed around the table. One brother played the sax, the other the drums. My sister, Pat, could sing. John, Bill, Peg, and Kate all played piano. I sometimes think it was Hugh's quiet mysteriousness that attracted me, his ability to be comfortable in silence. I always wondered what lay beneath the surface.

Late in the morning, two nurses help Hugh into a sitting position. It seems inconceivable to me that he can sit or stand, but he actually manages to balance on the bed. He tips right, steadies himself with both hands, pushes himself to his feet, and walks a few steps, dragging IVs with him. Immediately afterward, he falls asleep from the effort, or at least it appears that he is sleeping. It's hard to tell. His eyes have not been closing all the way the past two days. His lids, eerily cracked, make him look like he's spying. The nurse puts gel in his eyes to keep them lubricated.

Peggy stops by the hospital for an update and encourages the girls to come to dance again. "It will be good for you to get out of the hospital for an hour or two," she says. In an effort to rejoin the living, we head to Shuffles in the evening. The small shopping center parking lot is packed with minivans. Inside the dance studio, life bustles with bright painted murals, blaring music, and teenage energy. Mary suddenly leans up against me. "I don't think I want to dance, Mom," she says, looking pale. Anna runs to a vacant spot on the floor, smiling at her friends in the full-length mirror, and begins the warm-up while I steer Mary outdoors. The world outside of MCV feels contradictory to us—loud and happy—while we feel lonely and sad.

Out on the sidewalk, we stroll past Brunetti's restaurant arm in arm, and stop in the patch of grass at the end of the pavement for a minute. "Okay, Mary?" I ask.

"I'm thirsty. I just don't feel like dancing," she says.

"C'mon. We'll pick up a water bottle at Eckerd." We pass the noisy studio again, and the Atlee Library. On our way back to the Explorer, Mary asks if she can call her Aunt Kate. Lying across the back seat, she dials her cell phone and takes in Kate's voice. While they are talking, my oldest brother, Bill, calls me on my cell, so I leave the truck and sit down on the dirty sidewalk dotted with dried squished gum and candy wrappers. His deep, fatherly voice is an instant balm. Bill is the oldest of my siblings. He was often in charge when our parents were out. Now he's a successful lawyer and executive, a problem solver. He's been responsible and practical since the day he was born. Even the toddler pictures we have of him show his eyebrows furrowed in deep thought. He clears his throat, "Hello Rosemary, I was wondering how you're doing," he says.

"We're managing pretty well, Bill. It's hard, no news really." He asks about Hugh and the girls. After a short pause, he says, "I'm wondering how you are financially. Do you need any money? If you do, I can help out. All you need to do is say the word."

"So far, so good, Bill. But who knows later on. We are still getting vacation pay and his Human Resources department says he will be eligible for short-term disability soon. But it's great to know you're there if we need you."

"I love you, Rosie. Call my cell anytime. If you need me right away, call my assistant and she'll get hold of me. Give my love to Hugh and the girls too." As I snap my phone shut, I hold back tears and look up to the vast blue sky. I wish I could hug my big brother; I need the solid strength of him.

Money. How much do I owe so far? I hardly open my mail anymore. I let it sit three or four days before opening the envelopes, tossing most in the wastebasket. What remains is more work: bills to pay, insurance forms to complete. It piles up fast. "This is going to cost a fortune," the ICU nurse said. I haven't worked a corporate job since the girls were born. Working out of the house for a couple hundred dollars a week with no benefits will not support us. *Friggin money*, I think. *The root of all evil*, Pop used to say. I decide to call Ken's wife, the lawyer, and hear what she has to say.

With a deep breath, I collect myself and walk over to join Mary. She's still engaged in a long conversation with my sister. I lean against the sun-warmed body of the Explorer and try to calm my nerves, but I can't. This is the third time a family member has offered to give me money or pay for something. Do they all think we're broke? Hugh is certainly not working anytime soon, I'm not taking any jobs, and we're racking up bills by the minute. As a wave of panic rises in my throat, I swallow hard and decide not to think about it right now.

Mary waves to me, so I climb back in the van, and feel the setting sun warm me through the window. Promptly at seven, Anna comes skipping toward us with several friends who want to say hello to Mary.

The girls congregate around the parking lot in their jazz pants and leotards while I talk to Peggy. Mary's face animates around the edges as her friends surround her.

On our kiss-good-night visit to the hospital, Anna tells a drowsy Hugh about dance. "I can almost nail a triple pirouette, Dad! Want to see?" she says twirling. A lazy smile curls up on the right side of his face. Mary is quietly rubbing Hugh's feet to help him sleep. His first waking memory will be seeing Mary at the foot of his bed, her soft fingers kneading his arches.

Chapter 11

April 24, 2002

*Just wanted to let you know that my friend Ellen sends her love and is praying
for you all. Her little girl Madison is three and prays at night and at every meal
for God to take care of the man on the bicycle. Little hearts, big prayers.*

Love you all, Patty

- Patty King

Days 12-13

Mary and Anna have decided it is time to go back to school. They
have been out for eleven days. With tension and apprehension,
book bags that have not been unzipped for two weeks are emptied and
repacked. Drawer searches ensue for sharpened pencils and misplaced
calculators.

My six a.m. call to the nurse's station informs me that Hugh has
had a good night. His fever is down and his lungs are clearing up after
an infection, a common occurrence from lying flat for so long. Good
news to start the school day. "Butterflies?" I ask the girls as we head out
the door. Their heads nod, their bony shoulders sag under the weight
of heavy backpacks.

The girls and I walk through the wide front doors of Moody Middle
School. I always thought that was the perfect name for a middle school.
We part ways in the crowded hallway amid a swarm of students rushing
to beat the morning bell. Waving good-bye and turning away sharply is
all I can do to restrain myself from giving them an embarrassing mushy

sendoff before sending them into the world again. A short meeting with a guidance counselor assures me the teachers know Anna and Mary may need a little extra help to cope and catch up.

Anxious to reach the hospital, I stride down the now empty hallway, past the front office toward the main foyer. "Rosemary!" someone calls. I turn and see a realtor I know, a new acquaintance. "How are you? I heard about your husband. How awful!" she says while approaching.

"It is. I'm on my way to the hospital now. Thank you, but I need to run…"

"I know someone who was there at the scene, the day of the accident. She goes to my church. She's a registered nurse. She stopped to help your husband…"

"Oh my God," I interrupt, stunned at her news.

"She wants to talk to you. She would like to know he's okay."

I see Hugh hit the pavement in my mind. "I don't know," I mutter. "I guess."

We talk a few more minutes. She pulls a piece of scrap paper from her large bag and scribbles a name and phone number on it. "She's really nice. If you want to know about that day, call her anytime. I'll tell her I spoke to you. She'll be glad to know he lived through it."

While buckling my seatbelt and pulling away from the curb, I think about this witness, a nurse. I'm not sure I can stomach hearing all the graphic details of Hugh at the accident scene. I'm mostly curious about the woman that hit him. There has not been one word from her yet. Once I park at the hospital, I look again at the paper, fold it up into a small square, and place it snugly in my wallet for safekeeping.

Sitting next to Hugh's bed is comforting this morning. He is asleep after three straight days of being awake and pulling at tubes. Staring into his peaceful face, I can imagine he's my 'old' husband. But when he opens his eyes, he is not like my husband at all. It is the subtleness of a person, the shared secret smiles and intimate glances folded into the nuances of each encounter that create a relationship, and we have lost that connection. As he lies still, I talk to him about the girls' return to school and how nervous they feel but how brave they are being for us. It's a little like talking to myself. "They'll be alright," I assure him. "They have so many good friends and everyone is looking out for them." Hugh doesn't move. After digging around in my bottomless purse to find a pen, I begin to write in my journal. The pages fill up quickly.

Today is Hugh's sixth day out of the coma, and there is cause to celebrate. With help from his physical therapist, he pushes himself up from the bed, slowly takes a few wobbly steps and kisses me on the lips. This marks the first time he has made upright contact with me since the accident. It is not so much a romantic experience as a mechanical one, like receiving a stiff kiss from Frankenstein, complete with rigid arms and head scars, but he's moving and walking! To me, it's like watching him win the Tour de France. As soon as he's settled back in the bed, he says, "Again." Ah, now, there's the old Hugh shining through, I think.

In the afternoon, I have my first tour of the rehab center in the older section of the hospital on the second floor. I have to identify myself before being allowed to enter the heavy mechanized doors leading into the unit. Directly inside to the left is a nurse's station. On the right, patients congregate in wheelchairs or in plastic chairs, looking stranded, confused, or vacant. The air smells alternately of excrement and disinfectant making my overly full stomach lurch. I hope I've just hit it at the wrong time. "Hugh will progress rapidly here," says the director of the unit. The charge nurse introduces me to staff members before I'm shown the bedrooms, family meeting room, therapy rooms, dining room, and simulated kitchen where patients learn to perform simple cooking assignments in occupational therapy.

My shoulders tense into knots as I stand next to the nurse's station at the end of my tour and hear that Hugh may have to relearn the simplest of tasks. The director explains, "Hugh will work on toileting, walking, speaking, and planning as we go through our day. He'll also need to work on sequencing, doing things in order." It never occurred to me that Hugh could lose such basic skills as knowing the sequence to getting dressed—underwear before pants, socks before shoes—or knowing the activities required to groom himself each morning. He will also be evaluated in reading and writing. I will receive a report after he enters the rehab center. Papers are exchanged, signatures granted, and I shake hands cordially, as if the news I am hearing is not earth shattering. I am now officially Hugh's guardian. He is no longer my partner, he is my responsibility.

Late in the afternoon, my in-laws pick the girls up from school and drop them at the hospital for a visit. Down in the rehab center, I'm running late. My head swims with disturbing information. Glancing at my watch, I quickly excuse myself and dash to the lobby. No girls. We have missed each other on the elevator. I run the stairs two at a time to the eleventh floor, trying to beat them. I don't. I see them in the ICU standing beside Hugh without his cap on—his injured head visible— the chopped up oily pressed hair, gunk, staples, and tubes. Mary turns to me, her face bright pink. She bolts past me into the hall, crying. Her anguish explodes when I catch up to her, breathless but too late.

"Mom, you promised he'd have his cap on. I saw his head and I didn't want to see it!"

"Mary, I'm sorry, I had a busy day and didn't realize it..."

"Leave me alone!" she snaps and runs past me in tears, half stumbling. Still reeling from my trip to the Rehab Center, I let her go. I want to curl up in a ball right there in the hall and sob. Instead, I stand frozen, my face ashen. The ICU nurse grabs hold of my shoulders. "Rosemary, you can't create a happy version for her. She has to go through her own pain. You can't protect her from it. It's not your fault."

Anna takes my hand. "She'll be okay, Mom. She'll be back soon."

As I place the thin cotton cap carefully on Hugh's head, my jaws clench with repressed anger at the way all our lives are spinning wildly out of control. Moments later, a subdued Mary reappears, her face pale and gaunt. "Are you okay, Mary?" I ask, thinking to myself *what a stupid question* as the words leave my own mouth.

"I'm fine," she replies in a shrill voice. I think of the Aerosmith song that uses "Fine" as an acronym for "**F**ucked up, **I**nsecure **N**eurotic and **E**motional." That's us! We're all just FINE!

Concerned about the frazzled condition of my family, a nurse introduces me to a psychologist on staff who explains survivor counseling. I'm told the entire family can receive personalized help dealing with the many aspects of traumatic brain injury. Perking up at the idea, I say, "Girls, why don't we make an appointment and go talk to the counselor." Backs rigid, arms crossed, and eyes wide, they respond in unison, "Mom! That is *so* mental! Do you think we're *mental* or something?"

"Well, I know *I* am right now," I say a little louder than intended. I decide to go alone and see if I find it helpful before pushing Mary and Anna into something they clearly don't want to do. The following afternoon, I tentatively knock on the office door of the rehabilitative psychologist. We talk but I can't open up to her. I'm still too emotionally clogged. She hands me a book to read that looks as though it's written for a first grader. "This will help you communicate with your husband and help him deal with the consequences of the accident," she explains. I take the thin booklet from her and leaf through it. Like a coloring book, it's published in large print with pictures, and there is a workbook part for me to complete with Hugh. The questions read: "Why am I here?" "What's wrong with my memory?" "Who are all these people and why are they telling me what to do all the time?" Coloring book cartoons dot the pages. It's preschool. It's elementary. I feel insulted. I hate the book. I want to rip it into pieces. Besides, Hugh remembers us. I can't see why everyone thinks he's so impaired.

But the fact is: Hugh cannot remember things day to day. He has both retrograde amnesia (the inability to remember the accident and even several days before the accident) as well as post-traumatic amnesia (remembering only a few minutes or few hours ago, living in the now). Fully aware of this on some deep level, I am stuck in denial. It's a mental game I am playing, and a dangerous one, but I can't allow myself to know or admit that he is not going to return to me as he was ever again. Why didn't I know how much I loved him before? Why did I take him for granted so much of the time?

My drive home from the hospital is a blur. Somehow, I arrive in my own driveway. Instinct takes me up the steps, into the house, and to the bathroom, where I scrub my face before the girls arrive home from school. I sweep powdered blush on my cheeks to look alive for them.

Of course, Hugh's injury occurred on April 13th, and Hugh, a typical CPA, had not yet filed his tax return. Lee has generously offered to file an extension for us. I've also spoken to him about hiring a lawyer and he thinks I should. He has offered to drive the girls and me to the hospital for a goodnight visit with Hugh and we have a date to meet

Ken's wife, Liz. I also asked Jim and Kevin to attend to hear what she has to say.

Lee arrives at the house in the evening. He sorts through papers with me in Hugh's office while Anna and Mary finish eating dinner. Packing up his briefcase with a few manila folders and the townhouse rental checkbook, he turns to me smiling. "Well, the government won't be coming after you anytime soon. Ready to go to the hospital?"

By seven, the ICU is calm. The humming monitors create a repetitive symphony of swooshing and airbursts, the result of which is surprisingly meditative. Hugh is asleep.

"Hey Hugh, just stopping by to check up on you," Lee says. "Barbara says Hi too. I'm taking care of business for you while you rest. Don't worry about a thing." Lee turns to me in the hall when we're done visiting and says, "I admire Hugh's inner strength." Once Mary and Anna kiss Hugh goodnight, we all take the elevator to the lobby.

In the surgical waiting area of the cavernous main entrance we meet Liz, Kevin, and Jim. Liz is dressed in a navy business suit. Her white blouse is slightly untucked, and her skirt a bit rumpled from a long day at the office. But her voice is clear and strong. "I'm sorry you had to go through this, Rosemary," she says. "I have very little information, but I was able to get a copy of the police report." She pulls a paper from a file in her briefcase. "Would you like to see it?"

Trying to appear calm, I nod. Inside, I'm not so sure. I have been having trouble falling asleep. Every time I'm at rest, my mind relives the crash as I imagine it. I've replayed it in my mind a thousand times, each time a little different, because I don't have the real facts. I see Hugh being slammed, lying in the road unconscious.

Taking the paper, I read: "Patient's head went through windshield, came out and was knocked over car roof, denting roof, and trolling down the road." The words blur. I scan the document again: "eyes open, inappropriate words, combative…" I push the paper back at her, eyes full of tears. *He was awake, fighting.* I feel nauseated. *He was screaming.* I jump up from the electric jolt of this new information and gasp.

Mary and Anna sit nearby busy with homework. They glance over at me with worried looks on their faces. I send them my not-so-convincing *I'm okay* smile. Liz touches my shoulder. "I know it's hard. The way I see it, this woman was in the wrong," she says. "She clearly hit Hugh with the full front of her car. She had clear visibility and Hugh was where he should be. But I can tell you, Rosemary, this is going to be a long drawn out case. You will need a lawyer. It doesn't have to be me, but I strongly advise you get legal help."

After Kevin, Jim, and Lee ask her several questions, she hands me her business card. "This injury is devastating. Ken and I don't want to see your family suffer any more. Call me if I can help," she says while shaking my hand.

I hire her the next day and decide from this point on, I will gladly turn everything completely over to her while I focus on Hugh and the girls.

Chapter 12

Who or what is Jocko? It used to sit on your dad's bed...we would come to visit and every time, this monkey would be on the bed...I swore it never moved, and may never have been played with...but it was made of socks...the kind of old time hunting socks...they were kind of brown tweed with light beige toes...someone had made it for your dad. It had button eyes and sewn red lips...I've only known it as Jocko...I do not know if your dad named it or the person that gave it to him did, or maybe your grandmother did. I just know that Hugh made us think it was the only one in the world and of course, with that in mind, I wanted it, could not have it, and your dad had the only one. Therefore, he was lucky. Well, many years from then, I found a toy store full of Jockos and even though I was way too old to have one, I made sure that I bought one for my children whenever that would be. Last night, I went upstairs to the closet and took Jocko out of storage and he is sitting on the guest bed... hopefully he will bring that little extra hope that we all need to believe in.
Love, Aunt Betty
   - Betty O'Connell, Hugh's cousin and Krista's mother in Florida

Days 13-15

The toast won't pop.

Stalking the offending appliance, I pace with butter knife in hand. "Mom, just let it stay down the whole time instead of popping it up yourself!" chides Anna. I let out a huff and look away. There's too much to do today. Mary's knee has been hurting for weeks, but she has been hesitant to complain because she doesn't want to add to my worry list. She's already tried using anti-inflammatory meds, ice packs, and rest to no avail, so I finally took her to the doctor and he ordered her to physical therapy. After dropping Anna at school, I drive Mary over to her appointment.

I have not been an attentive mother lately and I know it. Consumed with the details of Hugh's recovery, I am in a world of my own most of the time. In a very real sense, Anna and Mary have lost both their parents over the past few weeks. Nerves are frayed, and the girls are constantly cued by relatives and friends to go easy on me. But what about them? As hard as I try to be the way I was with them before, energetic and engaged, I cannot. I am so grateful for every quiet moment they afford me, every free pass for a cranky mood, and every hug they offer.

"Done, Mom." Mary grabs up her school backpack from the waiting room and pauses for me at the door. Suddenly her smile looks so beautiful to me. I can see the incipient woman in her face.

"Mary, please let me know if that knee gets worse. I don't want you to think I'm too busy to help you with this." Of course I'm too busy, I tell myself, but what the hell, at least I can *sound* like a good mother.

Mary walks beside me with a limp. "I will, Mom. I'm not sure this therapy is helping much. It's not getting any better and they just keep doing the same things." We decide to finish this round of sessions and get another opinion if it doesn't improve.

"Ready for school?" I ask.

"Not really. I have another quiz today in geometry and I can hardly keep up," she says.

"Just do your best..." I begin but she cuts me off, "I know. I know, Mom." The rest of our ride to school is silent. I never say the right thing lately.

After leaving Mary at school, I'm surprised to see Hugh in his ICU cubicle seated in a chair, or rather, tied into the chair, so he won't get up and fall. A thick white strap across his waist restrains him like a high chair belt. His mother sits in a plastic chair inches from him, a curtain away from the next critical patient. Rita looks uncomfortable under the fluorescent lights; her features a mix of concern and forced pleasantness. There are no words to express her true thoughts, so she reverts to the weather as a topic of conversation. "It's a nice day outside today, dear," she says to Hugh. Thinking for a second in this small chamber of silence, she pauses, and then decides on a question, "How are you feeling today?"

No answer. Hugh stares vacantly at some far-off point, way beyond the curtain.

"I talked to your cousin, Betty, last night and she sends her love," Rita tries. After a few cursory attempts at small talk with little response, she signals her departure by pushing up on the arms of the chair. A flicker of recognition flashes in Hugh's eyes, and he suddenly remembers his good manners. Watching his mother intently, Hugh struggles to stand up with the chair tied to him. A slight smile creases her eyes. She tells him to sit and bends to kiss him on the cheek. "Work hard, Hugh. You're doing great. I love you," she says with her hands resting on his shoulders. He searches through round unblinking eyes for her as if trying to see more clearly. Her back is curved and the corners of her mouth droop, giving her a look of weary sadness. She lifts her large white pocketbook over her shoulder, and turns with a parting smile to her son. His head is tilted gently to one side. "Remember, work hard. I'm proud of you," she says as firmly as she can manage.

By April 26th, I'm told that Hugh is stable enough to be moved to the in-hospital Acute Brain Rehab Center, but there is not a bed available yet, so he is moved to the general medical/surgical floor in the interim. There is no personal nurse like the one who helped him around the clock in the ICU. This becomes an immediate problem. On Friday, the shift nurse reports that Hugh repeatedly pulled out his tubes and IVs. "Why are you doing this?" I ask him.

"Because the doctor told me to," he says in all seriousness.

"The doctor didn't tell you to pull that out!"

"Yes, he did," he responds, deadpan. His hand moves toward the IV again, but his eyes stay on me.

"Hugh, you are doing it again. That tube is for your medicine. I told you two seconds ago to leave that alone."

"You talk too much."

"You don't make any sense." *Tit for tat*, I think. *How old are we?*

The girls visit for an hour or two after school and still have time for friends at night, but I am exhausted in every way and still unable to sleep. My heart beats out of my chest every time I lie down. On

Saturday morning, aching from a fitful sleep, I stretch under the covers wishing I could fall back into the void of blissful nothingness and stay there until Hugh miraculously appears, healed. *Thank-you God for my daughters, my friends, this house, this bed, my brain* (I never gave thanks for my brain before). I'm reaching for gratitude—to think of what I have, rather than what's missing in life. *And, thank-you for Hugh. Does he know where he is? Why he's not home? Is he scared? Does he miss us?* I throw back my sheets and rouse the girls way before they are ready. "Time to go to the hospital," I say.

Entering Hugh's room ahead of Anna and Mary, I find him writhing in the bed, his hospital gown a thin rope twisted around his waist. He's completely exposed and reeking of filth. I quickly call a nurse and divert the girls to the hall for a few minutes while he is cleaned up. Since the floor is understaffed due to the shift change, I help the nurse move Hugh as she positions clean sheets, scrubs, and redresses him. The girls busy themselves with schoolwork, but they can probably overhear me say to the nurse, "He should not be on this unit yet. He needs more supervision. Don't you think this is dangerous?"

The nurse listens, but she's overworked and miffed as she confides that a few people called in sick last minute. "It's hard to get people late on a Friday night," she explains. "Today should be better. The full shift is expected."

The girls come back into the room feigning happy smiles for their father. "Hey Dad! How ya feelin?" Hugh shifts and yanks at the tubes protruding from his body.

As Mary sits cross-legged on the bed, she says, "Look at all these cards. Want me to read some to you?" While she tears open an envelope, Anna wrestles Hugh to keep him from ripping the IV out of his arm. After an hour, another nurse appears and asks us to take a break while she tends to a few of his needs. If we are not back when she's done, she'll secure his wrists to the bedrails. We can untie him when we return.

We travel eleven floors south to the cafeteria for a break, and when we return, Hugh is upright, swaying unsteadily by his bed, alone in the room. He has undone his own restraints, a trick he no doubt learned from his sailing days on the Great South Bay of Long Island. Looking our way, he wobbles precariously, gown askew, his eyes wild, like a disheveled bobble-head doll. Anna and Mary help me slowly settle him back into the large plastic recliner. After pushing him down a few times like a Jack-in-the-box, he's still agitated, so we help him onto the bed in hopes that soft pillows will keep him down. All engines seem to be firing at once today.

Two new quirky habits have emerged: shrugging and winking. Hugh's answer to almost any question is a distinctive "I don't know" shrug. To say 'yes,' he gives us a wink. He greets us with a husky, gritty voice that has no inflection. With his eyes popped unnaturally wide, he stares at our forms more in curiosity than recognition. We can see the moment it registers that we are the people he loves. A change comes over his face. I miss the easy body language we once shared; we could cruise through a conversation with few words based on our facial expressions and eye contact. "Come out! Come out! Wherever you are," I say, trying to be funny. Only it's not funny and I instantly regret it.

Once on the bed, Hugh is more talkative than usual. He says several short phrases to Anna that she writes in my diary, but mostly he keeps trying to make her pull out his IV. Mary eases herself onto the bed beside him and shows him pictures of people from work that have been sent by Hugh's assistant as greeting cards to jog his memory. "Dad, look at her. Do you know who she is?"

"Diane," he says, uninterested. Turning to his IV he grunts, "Can you pull it off? Can you untie my arm? Pull it out." Anna shakes her head no. "Scratch my nose." Anna scratches him.

Mary switches pictures. "Good, Dad," she says. "How about this one?" Her slim fingers frame another photo. Further agitated, Hugh raises his hand to the feeding tube in his nose and Anna swats it away. He lowers his hand and cunningly goes for the IV in his arm. Mary catches him this time. "Dad, don't do that," she cries. "The tube is there to help you." His persistence is wearing them out. Mary gently strokes his arm. "Leave it alone," she insists. "It's there for a reason."

Suddenly, Hugh has had enough. He summons up a dominant paternal voice and orders her to take the tube out now. She shakes her head *no*. Glaring at her, he snarls, "If you won't help me, then GO!" Mary rushes from the room in tears.

He then turns on Anna, but she fires back at him, mad over the encounter with her sister, "Fine, Dad! Go ahead and pull all the stupid tubes out! See if I care!" She backs up to the wall, slides down and wraps her arms around her knees, biting back her tears; they pool up and stream down her face anyway.

We all know that Hugh has no idea what he is saying and doing, but it doesn't make it any easier to accept that he's behaving like an unreasonable child in an overgrown body. We all want this part to be over. Hugh is awake, moving, and talking—yet not with us at all. For two teenage girls it is devastating. Why does their dad have to be this way? Betty's email echoes in my mind. "Who or what is Jocko?"

Who or what is Hugh?

Like Jocko, he sits alone on the bed. He is unique. Years later Betty realizes that there is a whole toy store full of Jockos that she never knew existed. The girls and I have come to understand that there is a whole other reality for many people that we never thought about before, the ragged stranger we scurry past because he seems dangerous and disturbed, those we watch from a distance and avoid because they are wild eyed and talking to themselves. Those we judge—that strange man, that odd woman. What had they gone through that we had ignored? Were they once happy healthy people who suffered an accident? Never again will we dismiss these people or fail to utter a prayer on their behalf.

I summon the nurse. She feeds Hugh some medicine and ties his wrists to the bedrail. Too sad to watch, the girls and I trudge back to the car and on comes Hugh's Bon Jovi CD playing "Two Story Town." We all sing along with the chorus and begin to shout out our tension with the double-edged lyrics:

It's the same old shit going around
I'm going down, down, down, down, down

Screaming the refrain together feels like busting out of an emotional prison. We replay it and sing louder, then laugh in a giddy frenzy until we fall silent as we pull into our driveway, surprised to see visitors in our yard. Kevin's wife, Donnelle, is mowing the lawn on the John Deere with her two year old, Caleigh, snug on her lap. Kevin and Rick are raking up sticks and leaves and Jim is busy mulching the gardens.

They came to do a spring-cleaning and the only thing I have to offer them is a cold drink and a troubling update. Kevin gulps down some ice water while Caleigh skips along the sidewalk. "This stage is temporary Rosemary," he says. "He'll come around soon." Donnelle shoots me a look of connection. She knows, I think. She knows how frightened I am. And just her look makes me feel a little less isolated.

Alone with Hugh in the evening, I rotate his arms above his head to keep his limbs flexible. It feels better to do something physical with him than to try to relate verbally. As I stretch his arms up, I search his eyes for recognition. Not much seems to register and he won't converse. I stay with him as long as possible so he remains untied. Afterward, Debbie Willis brings Amanda over to spend the night with the girls. Although I smile and joke as usual, she senses my mood, and stays to talk with me for a while.

Settled on the sofa, she inquires, "It sounds like Hugh is making some progress. He's got a lot of help in the hospital, but how are you doing these days?"

"I'm wiped out. I feel helpless and I don't have any idea when he'll be himself again. Now a speech therapist is getting involved to do a swallow study to see if he can get the feeding tube removed. Then they'll set him up for speech therapy in rehab."

"How long will he have to be in the hospital?"

"I'm not sure. No one's really said yet. He still hasn't even gotten to rehab—the rehab unit in the hospital, I mean. But there's a lot to think about. All these stairs—I don't know where he's going to rest down here when he comes home. The couch is too low. My parents gave me money for a recliner but I don't have time to shop for furniture."

"I'll find a recliner! You know I'm always shopping. Hecht's is having a sale that I can check out for you. Jeff can test the size, he's tall like Hugh." Debbie smiles and wraps me in a warm hug. I thank her at the front door for helping me so willingly. "Anytime," she says.

Before dawn on Sunday, I begin compiling a notebook of personal information about Hugh for the nurses and doctors to use in rehab. I include a timeline of his life events, his food preferences, and pictures of family and friends that he can identify. It also outlines the sports he participated in (competitive sailing, surfing, swimming, cycling, and triathlons) and some details that could be used when questioning him about his past for therapy. Assembling this book helps me connect again with Hugh. By writing down his life I am validating his past. I want so much to jump into that past. I want my husband back.

Chapter 13

I am out and about driving somewhere every two hours. I would love to pick up the girls or take them to places if needed or even downtown... PLEASE take care of your own needs and bodies before any others so that you all will be there for Hugh when he arrives at his front door. You owe no one an explanation about not writing or calling...Family first!
Love to you all...will be there for the many months ahead,
Nancy

-Email from Nancy Hendrickson

Days 16-18

Rick calls early on Sunday morning to see if anyone needs a ride to the hospital since he and Lara will visit in the afternoon. I quickly accept his offer to shuttle the girls. I'm extra quiet as I lock the door behind me so I don't wake them up, glad that they can sleep in for a change.

When I arrive at Hugh's hospital room, I notice the hard, plastic helmet on his raw head is fastened under his chin around the neck brace, making him wince. I ask the nurse for the third time if we can do something about the helmet situation. Mary called me out on my *pestering* earlier in the week. "Mom, why do you have to bother everyone at the hospital all the time?"

"I'm not bothering them. I always ask in a nice way," I had told her. "I'm advocating for Dad because he can't ask for things himself right now." She crossed her arms over her chest, which made me continue,

"Look, I'm fine if he wears it when we're not here, but when we're with him, it's not necessary, and it clearly hurts."

Hugh is active this morning. He shuffles to the nurse's station and back with slow steps, dragging his IV pole in his longest walk yet. He still continually grabs for his feeding tube and I continually stop him. Many times, I discover too late that he's just putting his hands to his face to scratch a spot, but I don't trust him anymore, so he's not even afforded that small measure of relief. I'm thankful that Hugh has not turned violent or obscene, but I wish he could verbalize what he wants and needs. His persistence is maddening.

The girls call my cell phone to tell me not to eat lunch because they made me a healthy lunch they will bring to the hospital. As I flip my phone shut, Dr. Ward stops in on his rounds. As a last resort I tell him I think the helmet is painful for Hugh. He orders the helmet off Hugh's head for the time being. Every time I see that man I want to hug him for something. When Dr. Ward is about to leave, he sees me peeling Hugh's fingers from the food tube again. "See if you can get him to eat something so we can pull that tube out for good," he says with a smile.

Spurred along, I open up a container of yogurt from the food tray. "How about a spoonful, Hon. It's strawberry—your favorite." Seeing that Hugh is not interested, I switch tactics and treats. I lift a can of Boost before his eyes with my hand obscuring the label, and in a perky voice I say, "Here, Hugh, try a sip of this, it tastes like a vanilla milkshake." The liquid is a beige-gray color. He barely dips his tongue in the can before thrusting it back at me with a scrunched-up face. "You have it," he says. My credibility now shot, I roll the tray away.

Rick and Lara have dropped the girls off. Each one is carrying a part of my healthy lunch: fresh fruit and cut-up veggies. While I munch on a carrot stick, Electra peeks her head in, sneaks up behind me, and rubs my neck—one of the strong perks of friendship with a masseuse. Her trained fingers plow into the tops of my shoulders. She talks to me while working out a knot, "There is enough pent up stress in this little neck to fuel a missile. Try some Advil and ice when you get home. Your neck must hurt."

Hugh's parents shuffle in next. Rita hands me a bar of Ghirardelli dark chocolate. "Isn't this the kind you love?" she asks. I quickly abandon the carrot stick for the candy. Anna shoots me a disapproving smirk while Mary playfully taunts, "You can have that after you eat your broccoli!" Rita grins, happy to have stirred up a silly controversy with indulgence.

Late in the afternoon, a new nurse stops in and introduces herself as a personal friend of Larry Piper, Hugh's old cycling coach from his racing days. He now owns his own medical consulting company that focuses on medical litigation. She's come to send Larry's regards and see if there is anything on the medical end she can do to make life a little easier.

Not expecting miracles, I say, "Hugh has a bad back. I hate to see him tied to the bed all night unable to stretch out or roll over." She nods in understanding as I continue, "The last thing I want is for his back to go out. I keep asking him how his back feels but, he can't answer me coherently, so I don't know if it's bothering him or not." Mary looks at the ceiling as if to say, "Can you think of anything else to ask for, Mom?" Anna stifles a laugh.

The nurse thinks for a second. "Let me look into something. I think I have an idea but I have to check it out," she says. She purposefully strides out of the room, returning a short while later looking pleased. "We have a night sitter program. The hospital can pay to have a person stay with Hugh so he won't have to be restrained. This way he can move around, but won't get out of bed and hurt himself. Give me your home number."

Not long after we arrive home at night, she calls. "The night sitter will be here starting tomorrow and will come every night that Hugh's on this unit," she says.

"Has anyone told you today that you are an angel, an absolute living saint?" I say, feeling a huge weight lift off my chest.

"No," she says. "But I'll work hard to live up to the nicknames you give me!"

I fall asleep at night without a pill and wake up unusually clearheaded for a Monday morning.

"If you go to the store today, could you get some apples?" Mary asks as she jumps out of the van in front of school. Anna chimes in, "I like apple sauce better. Can you get the snack size? Not the cinnamon one!"

"I'll try to remember," I yell to them as they run across the lawn toward the front entrance. Upon arrival at the hospital, Hugh's R.N. reports that he has finally pulled out his feeding tube one time too many, so she will leave it out and send him for a swallow study. Score one for Hugh. He passes. If he eats, they will keep it out. Now he only has the IV's in his arm and the neck brace to contend with. He switches focus to the neck brace, his new archenemy.

Eating and drinking are now foreign to Hugh. He's like a caveman who curiously inspects his food and makes a sour face as he pushes it away in disgust. His new pastime is struggling to get the collar off his neck. It's the hard plastic type that makes it uncomfortable for him to swallow with his chin pointing up. The doctors say that as soon as he can cooperate enough for a flex and extension x-ray, they will check his neck and see if it can come off. He pulls at the collar constantly. No explanation placates him because he can't remember what I explained five minutes ago. I gently take his hand and place it on the armrest of his chair. After he attempts several more times, I grab his hand, squeeze it, and firmly place it on the armrest in exasperation. It's like training a toddler. He looks up at me as I press his hand down for the fifteenth time.

"Why?" His expression is a mix of innocence and aggravation.

"Because you are in the hospital and it's the rules."

"You worry too much about the rules," he says in his brain-injured James Dean way.

"Hugh, you could hurt yourself. That brace is there to protect you."

He looks right through me as his hand comes up again. His tenacity intact, he says, "Just take it off and don't worry about the rules," as if this is some elementary rule and not one that can affect his spinal health.

"Stop it. Just stop it, Hugh. Leave the collar alone!" I try to sound authoritative even though it's not in my nature to be forceful. Our encounters are no longer husband and wife exchanges but something completely different. When I say, "I love you," he says, "I love you too," then slides back into his android state. It's as if he's displaying a programmed response rather than an emotion. I wish I could reach deep down inside him and physically pull his spirit back out. Holding his face in my hands I say, "I love you so much. Do you know that?"

"Take it off," he says, deadpan.

The physical therapist and a nurse arrive to help Hugh stand. He quickly grows irritated with them. The PT is a tall, solid woman. She and the nurse each take one arm as she instructs him exactly how to move. "Here you go, Mr. Rawlins, use your arm to push up." Hugh gives her a dirty look.

"Let go of me," he says, wiggling away, "I can do it." The therapist tells him she has to hold on to him, it's the hospital's rule. His face hardens again at the word *rule*. I watch in amusement as he grudgingly works with them, cooperating only because it's two against one.

Hugh eats a few bites of a peanut butter and jelly sandwich and two chocolate teddy grahams—maybe all of fifty calories. He is noticeably thinner since the accident, and has had next to nothing to eat since the food tube came out. I don't know how he can be so obstinate with no caloric energy! He looks right in my eyes as he tries to wrench the collar off, challenging me to stop him. He sees that I am shaking my head "no" and pulls the collar anyway in defiance. Finally, he manages to yank it off when I am otherwise occupied, but his victory is short-lived; a nurse rushes in and wraps white surgical tape around his neck to seal the Velcro even tighter. Within minutes after she leaves, he rips through the tape in just a few swipes. Like a frustrated sibling, I tell on him. The exasperated nurse then warns him, "You do that one more time and your hands will be restrained again." He forgets the warning within minutes and I am back at him, pushing his hands away from the neck brace.

After repeatedly leaning over to stop him, I finally stand up, stretch my back, and let out one of my stress-releasing drawn-out sighs. As I exhale, I hear his old voice in its exact familiar intonation say, "What's wrong honey?" Eyebrows raised, he looks inquisitively around the room for whatever it is that could be irritating me. It is the sweetest moment, such a familiar encounter with such a typical response.

"Nothing, Hugh," I answer. "What could be wrong?" I burst out laughing as he looks at me like I'm nuts. He doesn't even know that he is the object of my frustration. He goes back to pulling at the neck brace again. "God Almighty, give me strength," I mutter, and he looks at me again curiously.

The food trays continue to arrive and are returned to the kitchen untouched. Once in a while I eat Hugh's lunch to justify paying for it, but I prefer my usual diet of ice water and dark chocolate. It's rather hypocritical of me to be so concerned about Hugh's diet right now when I'm dropping pounds from living on semi-sweet squares and high-caffeine coffee. I am told his aversion to food is a common occurrence after having a food tube and that he will gradually regain his appetite and begin to eat.

All this talk about food has made me think I should buy some decent food for our house and try to get back on track with better eating habits. I tiptoe away, leaving Hugh half asleep on the bed, and head to Ukrop's Supermarket. I intentionally park on Linguine Lane so I can find my car when I'm done. The girls are beginning to call me Mrs. Magoo. On a recent shopping trip I was so engrossed in my thoughts, people swerved away from me like fleeing minnows as I meandered about the grocery aisles in a dreamlike state. Anna cautioned me repeatedly, "Mom, watch where you're going, you almost ran into that old lady."

I just smiled at her and said, "But I didn't, did I?"

She shook her head. "You missed her by a millimeter! I don't know how you do it!" On another trip, I was so distracted it took me over ten minutes to find my car in the parking lot. That's when I decided that Linguine Lane is where I'll always park.

The girls arrive home to the smell of food cooking: pasta with tomato sauce for the girls, and pesto for me. "Wow, Mom, are you cooking?" Mary asks. Wide smiles fill their faces.

"Yes, and I'm really going to try to keep more healthy stuff in the house from now on. Thanks, girls, for getting me started. Want to start chopping stuff for salads?" I ask.

Anna opens the fridge and pulls out lettuce, carrots, a cucumber, and tomato. Mary is stooped over the stove smelling and tasting. "Mom, can we make homemade chicken tenders soon?" Mary asks.

"Sure. Let's do that tomorrow." The phone rings and it's Lara, Rick's wife. She tells me the story of a visit she and Rick had when the girls and I were not there. She says when they entered Hugh's hospital room, she sensed that Rick was emotionally overwhelmed, so she decided to talk a little. Hugh's eyes were closed and there was no reaction from him as she spoke. Then Rick whispered, "Hey Hugh," and Hugh moved, as if recognizing Rick's voice. He reached out his hand. Rick took Hugh's hand to shake it, and Hugh gripped it tight. Lara said they just stood there, hands locked in friendship for several minutes, and that lingering handshake was one of the most beautiful moments she had ever witnessed.

Lost in her story, I jump at the sound of the smoke alarm. I burned the garlic bread.

Chapter 14

Hugh,
You have so much to "get better" for! Keep fighting! We love you.
Scott, Kelly, Blake and Davis

-Kelly King's Family

Days 19-23

Hugh is transferred to the Acute Brain Rehabilitation Center in MCV Hospital on Wednesday, May 1st. He is now in another wing, downstairs. He has traveled from the fourth floor ICU, to the eleventh floor general surgery, to the second Floor Acute Brain Rehab in eighteen days. All new staff again. This time it's even more confusing; there are ten people involved in his care: two rehab doctors (the Director of Rehab and a resident); his surgeon, Dr. Ward; a neuropsychologist; a nurse; physical therapist; occupational therapist; recreational therapist; speech therapist; and social worker. I buy a French bulletin board, hang it by my phone, and immediately plaster every inch of it with medical business cards for easy access.

Hugh is put on two meds: Ritalin, which is said to increase attention in adults, even though it's used to relax hyperactive children, and Zoloft. When I ask the rehab doctor: "Why is he on Zoloft? Isn't that for depression?" he responds, "Yes. We just assume he will be depressed when he comes around. It pretty much goes with the territory. The Zoloft will help." This sums it up for me: Hugh's condition is so bad, how could he *not* be depressed?

On the day Hugh is transferred, a doctor I had met in the ICU who had a personal experience with brain injury in his family greets me in the hall. He is not involved in Hugh's care but he's concerned. He confides to me that his loved one had attempted suicide a year after her stroke. With compassion, he cautions me, "You're in this for a very long time. It's going to be physically and emotionally demanding, so you better take care of yourself. Caring for the brain-injured is a marathon, not a sprint. Has anyone told you about rehab yet?"

"A little," I answer, taken aback at his frankness, but hungry for the truth.

"You look tired," he says. The phrase "No shit, Sherlock" comes to mind, something Hugh used to say. He rarely cursed in anger, but had a few standard lines like that one.

"I am tired, but I want to be here all the time," I say.

"Why? Why do you think you need to be here all the time?"

"I feel guilty if I'm not here. What if he needs me?"

"Of course he needs you, but not all the time. Rosemary, you need to go on with your life. He's fine in here. He's doing the work he needs to do to get better. You need to get things ready at home, give the kids some attention, and catch up on your own life. Now is a good time. Hugh will be kept extremely busy in his therapies and when they are done with him, I guarantee, all he will want to do is sleep. Go home and get some rest. Visit in the evening with your girls. You'll need your strength when he gets home."

He walks along beside me as I head to the unit and tells me a story about a muscle-bound football player who was once on this ward. His only injury was a traumatic brain injury. "He was a two-hundred-fifty-pound hulk begging for his second serious accident. This guy would run down the long hall and yell, 'Tackle!' and believe it or not, none of these nurses or aides ever got hurt." Pointing at the nurses through the window of the double doors, he assures me, "If these people can take care of *that* football player, they can take good care of your husband."

"I'm sure," I say, while simultaneously thinking *I can take better care of him.*

"One more thing," he continues, "I would recommend restricting visitors in rehab to six or seven close relatives or friends. He will benefit from that—get the rest he needs." Grasping my elbow, he says, "You stay well now."

Outside the Brain Rehab entrance, we part ways. "Thank you, doctor. I'll try," I promise. "You do the same." My weak smile earns a perceptive look from the doctor. *He's been me,* I think. *He knows what I'm thinking.* I ring the buzzer and show identification to get in. As instructed on my tour, I check the large dry erase board that spells out the schedule for each patient each day. Hugh's due in the dining room. Round tables in this room hang down from the ceiling like huge spiders with their long legs touching at the top. No table legs touch the floor; this way all the wheelchairs can easily slide under. Hugh isn't there.

Walking back to the nurse's station, I observe how each patient's condition varies in severity. There are some in halos, some in wheelchairs; others are walking, but almost all look bewildered. Family members sit with their loved ones looking dazed and gaunt. A thirty-something woman is leaning forward in her wheelchair, dressed in a stained snap-up smock, her crooked arm curled into her chest. Her dirty hair, matted in strings, hangs down the side of her face like a beaded curtain. She is trying to look up at her husband, an overemphatic smile plastered on her face. Her husband sits numbly by her, his hands in his lap, face glazed over in exhaustion and hopelessness. My heart refuses to take this in. I march ahead.

"I'm looking for Hugh Rawlins," I say to the nurse at the circular desk. She points me down the hall. Each room has a little flag hanging outside it with a picture on the flag, so patients can find their room by the picture. "He's in the yellow dog room," she says.

I spot a mini banner with a white lab's happy face on it and walk in. It's a semi-private room. In the first bed is a tall thin man with a sign on his bed that reads: *My name is Ron. I had a stroke. I don't speak yet.* Hugh's curtain is drawn; he has the window bed. A TV hangs from the ceiling in the middle of the room so both people can watch. Each patient has a remote, but they sit untouched. This will be fun, I think as I remember how my husband loves control of the remote. I visualize a TV war—one TV, two men. I quickly see that I'm worrying for nothing. They're both passed out.

In his cramped section of the room, Hugh is sprawled across the mattress, asleep on top of his covers. I'm told he will not be allowed out of bed until he has a Doppler test to see if he has any blood clots in his legs from lying down so long. The test is scheduled for the afternoon. I sit by him, lean over for a kiss, in hopes that he'll wake up, but he snorts and returns to dreamland, so I organize clothing in the dresser. As instructed, I brought athletic type clothes that will be comfortable and easy to put on: sweats, socks, sneakers and pajamas. He needs seven full outfits like this, so I will need to go shopping. Hugh becomes attached to certain articles of clothing and wears them until they are threadbare. He's yelled at me in the past for throwing out t-shirts with gaping holes in them. Air conditioning, he calls it. All of a sudden, new athletic wear sounds like a good idea.

Every personal item has to have his name on it. Since he will be more active in rehab, he has to wear a helmet. I ask the rehab people to fit him with a new one. They take head measurements and assure me the newer helmet will not be as tight as this first one. Hugh sleeps soundly through my entire visit, which makes me think of the doctor's words: do I really need to be here? I make small talk and he sleeps through it. Sometimes I say ridiculous things to get a response just for fun, like: "Hey Hugh, there's a huge black beetle on your nose!"

Snore. I want to see his old expressive face—any expression other than that blank look. He is more interested in sleeping just now. "Okay, be that way," I whisper like a rejected child.

Patty King picks the girls up from school and drops them at the hospital entrance. She calls my cell. "Hi Hon," she says. "The girls are here—they're just getting out of my truck—call me if you need anything else!"

I meet Anna and Mary in the lobby and show them the way to Hugh's new room—different wing, different elevator, down instead of up. The bedroom is crowded, so we vie for the one comfortable chair. "The biggest butt wins," I say, and take the prize. The girls climb onto the bed with Hugh. He stirs and wakes up, smiles at the girls, but he's groggy. We can't stay long since it's a dance night. On the way out, the girls say they're starving. "Can we grab a hot dog at Jonathan's cart?" they ask—so much for the healthy meal program. While they dance at

Shuffles, I treat myself to dinner at Brunetti's next door. Alone at the table, I pretend to read.

The following morning, I take the doctor's advice after a nurse informs me that Hugh will be in back-to-back therapies all morning. I wake up and see the girls off to school. In my own house alone for the first time in weeks, I put on a pot of coffee, throw in some laundry, sort through paperwork, and call the nurse's station to check on Hugh. I slap together a peanut butter and jelly sandwich for him, silently hoping I won't be throwing it out later, and arrive at the hospital by eleven o'clock in the morning, refreshed.

As I enter the unit, I see Hugh in his wheelchair outside the nurse's station beaming. He has just had another CT scan, and his neck is fine. His collar is coming off today! The nurses let him remove it himself and he tears it off enthusiastically. I can hardly contain my excitement. After he hands it to me triumphantly, I look up at his nurse, and she smiles with tears in her eyes.

"Why are you crying?" I ask her.

"Because *you* are so happy," she says, staring at me as if she's witnessing a transformation. I realize that I look as gaunt as the other visitors I have noticed. I have dropped over ten pounds in two weeks. Stress and nervous energy quickly burn up every bite I eat; my stomach churns like a cement mixer the minute food hits it. At 5'5", I am down to 115 pounds. I haven't seen that weight in years.

I have been asked to participate in physical therapy with Hugh and his PT to learn how to help him when he comes home. Hugh can walk, but his balance is severely affected and his inability to focus and concentrate makes it dangerous for him to be out walking alone. The therapist shows me his gait belt, a thick canvas strap that ties around his waist to guide and balance him if he should begin to sway. I'm told the gait belt will be an absolute necessity every time Hugh gets up for the next three months until he has his bone flap replaced—the section of his skull that was removed. I cannot help but think of the gait belt as a leash.

My husband is on a leash.

He also has his new helmet, a real eyesore—thick, bright white plastic with a red, white, and blue strap. At least it is not as tight as the last one and has soft pads inside. The helmet has to be on his head even if he is sitting, we are told, no exceptions. It looks like a huge white gumball on his head.

Hugh's PT patiently teaches me to walk beside Hugh holding onto the gait belt and using it only to guide, not to pull. Then she teaches me strategies to go up and down stairs. She also teaches Hugh how to get up on his own if he does fall. This is difficult due to general weakness and the significant loss of his left side. He's instructed to get on all fours, try to pull himself up on a chair or other low piece of furniture with me spotting him, and then stand. His weak left arm makes him look like a three-legged dog. After our joint session, he is led into speech therapy.

I begin to realize why I have been told to take time out. The rehab center keeps Hugh busy, and he is less focused when I'm around. In fact, I'm a distraction to everyone. I'm not trained to deal with him like the nurses and therapists. Shamefully, I feel jealous of how well they interact with him. Feeling like an outsider with my own husband, I melt into the background and do little except sit in the hallway with the other patients, my pocketbook in my lap, waiting for brief intervals to see him move from therapy room to therapy room. If I'm trying to stay out of the way, why don't I just stay away?

At mealtime, I want to eat lunch with Hugh, but even meals are part of his treatment plan. A therapist leads him to the table in his wheelchair. One quick glance at his food tray and he backs away quickly, turning his right wheel while scooting his feet. His lifeless left hand sits in his lap. I sit in the background watching. "It's lunchtime, Mr. Rawlins. Come and eat," the therapist prompts. She tries to feed him like a two-year old or coax him to eat himself. He has no attention span and wheels himself in circles or from one end of the room to the other, crazy in love with the wheels on the chair. Barely any food makes it into his mouth. Hugh has lost over thirty pounds, and acts as if his body does not register hunger anymore. I grow frantic watching him refuse to eat.

The next day, I deliver a goody bag filled with peanut butter sandwiches, power bars, and other small food items he used to eat. I write down his favorite foods, and tape notes to brown bags, hoping the nurses will tempt him with these when I'm gone.

One morning, I discover that an aide has tried to get Hugh to eat scrambled eggs. Hugh has always hated eggs, so I hang up a poster that reads: NO EGGS FOR HUGH RAWLINS. I'm afraid he'll eat nothing if forced to eat the things he hates. My logical mind knows the nurses are telling jokes about my being a control freak. I feel stupid, but I can't stop myself. To their credit, they never make any remarks in my presence and let me hang my posters, knowing that it makes me feel better. In truth, I feel useless and pathetic.

Like living bruises, purple clouds churn in the sky. Severe thunderstorms and a tornado warning blare on the radio in the evening. Mary has arranged for a ride to a meeting to plan her school trip to Spain for the coming summer. Anna had gone to France the previous summer with students. We had them take their foreign language trips in separate years so we could afford it. I'm not sure it's wise to spend this money now, but I can't bring myself to tell Mary she can't go. The trip is well discounted and we had planned for it.

My phone rings after Mary leaves. It's Terry calling from Vermont. "Oh my God, Rosemary, I just heard about the tornado warning. It's going to hit your house! You have the worst luck of anyone I know." We laugh but she's only half-kidding. As the rain beats down in torrents on the deck, my mind spins disaster scenarios about Mary, who is in someone's car. I go from zero to100 in seconds when it comes to imagining danger: poor visibility, sliding cars, hydroplaning, head on collisions. "Mom, are you okay?" It's Anna watching me look out the back window.

"Yeah, but look at this storm. Mary just left," I say, alarmed.

"We always have storms. She'll be alright," she says with a tone that adds *and you are so weird lately!*

By the end of Hugh's first week in the acute brain rehab, the constant stress is making me feel sick and run down. I make an appointment to see my family doctor. Rifling through my purse for the flimsy insurance card that always gets lost in my wallet, I grab the car keys just as the doorbell rings. Standing on the front porch is Lawrence Liesfeld, the man who built our house two years ago. Shifting his feet from side to side as he pours out his concern for the family, he tells me about a relative of his own who suffered a brain injury. "I know how hard this can be," he says. "You'll need some changes 'round the house." Stepping into the foyer, he runs his hand along the wall envisioning aloud the changes he could make. "Here, we could put in handrails, then build a stall shower where the entrance to the garage is. This way, we could tear it all down when Hugh is well again, and your house will still look like new." I can barely get a word in edgewise.

"And don't you worry none either; this won't cost you a cent. I've already talked to a few friends and we have donations from local stores. Everyone wants to help," he says earnestly. "Here in Virginia, we take care of one another." My eyes well up instantly. Lawrence smiles as he pulls away in his truck, sending me off with a friendly wave as I rush off to my doctor appointment, basking in unexpected generosity and the basic goodness in people.

My family physician greets me warmly. "What's the trouble?" He knows about Hugh's accident from the hospital.

"I think I'm having a heart attack. I'm having frequent chest pains and sometimes they don't go right away." The doctor checks me over.

"Rosemary, you look fine. It's caused by stress. Look what's been going on in your life." I sit on the examining table, searching him for a magical cure. "Your pressure is fine, heart sounds good," he reassures me.

"But I'm scared to death of these chest pains. My father had a heart attack when he was only fifty-five. What if something happens to me? I have no back-up. What about the kids?"

"Whoa! Wait a minute. Nothing is going to happen to you," the doctor says while holding up his hand. We discuss my anxiety; he decides it's in the normal range for the circumstances and I don't need an anti-anxiety or anti-depressant drug. After a series of questions, he nods sympathetically and says, "Unfortunately, it's true what they say about a broken heart. It actually does hurt. That's what's bothering you, but you are handling things very well, considering." I recall my father's cardiologist saying: "You're in pretty good shape for the shape you're in!" I guess that should be my line now.

The doctor sits on the round rolling chair and drafts up a script to refill my Ambien. "You do need to sleep, so make sure you get some rest," he advises. I can't help thinking that *rest* is not what I usually get these days; it's more like drug-induced oblivion, but heck, whatever works. At least he's convinced me that I won't drop dead anytime soon.

Before driving to the hospital, I stop by the Kroger pharmacy. Joe, my pharmacist asks, "How is Mary's knee coming along? How is Hugh these days?"

"Joe, the whole family is falling apart. So far Anna's the only one not on prescription drugs, but she said her throat hurt this morning, so who knows…"

"Aw, maybe it's just allergies, Rosemary. At least let's hope so," he smiles.

Grabbing up a few more items, I whisper across the counter, "I feel like an idiot, I went to the doctor thinking I was having a heart attack and he says it's only stress." Dramatically sifting through a pile of chocolate I just placed next to my sleeping pills, he says, "Or it's all this chocolate giving you heartburn!"

"Ooh! Don't take my chocolate away. I'll keep the heartburn. Ring that up and throw in some Rolaids, would you? Thanks, Joe!" He shakes his head at me as I walk out of the store into the parking lot thinking about the word *stress*. It's such an overused word. I used to say I was stressed out if I was late for an appointment. Now I know what it really means. I wonder if the doctor thinks I'm crazy, but then I hear Hugh's voice telling me to stop analyzing everything. He used to ask me all the time, "Why do you worry about what everyone else thinks? Who cares as long as you're happy?"

"But I'm not happy. I miss you," I murmur into the empty car.

It is late morning already. The recreational therapist asks if I'd like to join her with Hugh on a mini field trip out of the unit and up to the lobby on a quest to buy a candy bar from the machine. "Would you like to buy your wife some candy, Mr. Rawlins?" she asks. This, apparently, is considered a major cognitive exercise. Hugh is sitting in his wheelchair, strapped in with his gait belt and wearing his helmet. "Yes," he nods without much emotion.

Hugh wheels himself, using his feet without the footrests to propel the chair, following the detailed instructions of the therapist. When he counts out two quarters at the candy machine, she says, "Good, Mr. Rawlins, let's put it in the machine." I am trying to look engaged and excited by this amazing feat.

Hugh looks up at me, his face radiating sincerity, "What do you want?" he asks. The tone in his voice softens my heart.

"Gum," I reply. We smile at each other like two strangers drawn together by some mysterious force. It takes a few minutes to review how to push the corresponding button for a pack of gum.

Hugh points and asks, "B12?" The therapist shakes her head side-to-side. Hugh keeps looking at her to confirm the right button. He is directed to look at the letters and numbers that match where the gum is placed. As he stares at the machine, his breathing becomes more rapid. Glancing from the machine to us for approval he finally pushes button C6, and out comes the gum. He hands it to me and stretches his neck for a kiss. I deliver one promptly. When it's time to go back, he looks around the massive lobby past the candy machines and sees hallways, the bustling front entrance, people sitting, people chatting, people rushing by...people, people, people. Overwhelmed, he shuts down, his face suddenly blank.

The therapist is not deterred. "First, we will look for the hallway with the elevators," she prompts. He sees the sign and begins wheeling. With constant reminding, we travel back to the Rehab unit where Hugh falls asleep the minute he climbs into bed. This twenty-minute trip and the exhaustive concentration it took for him to complete it has knocked him flat.

Hugh's parents meet him for lunch while I run errands. "Hugh ate all the homemade applesauce I made him. I'm whipping up another batch," Rita tells me on the phone. Encouraged, the girls and I decide we'll pick up hamburgers and try to eat dinner with Hugh in the family room at the hospital. The room is carpeted with two couches and a table for four, as homey as a room in a hospital can be. We position ourselves around the table and the girls motion for Hugh to join us as they set the table. Hugh wheels himself back and forth and in circles; he races toward the wall, stops short and turns. When the girls get up to lure him over, he gestures "After you," with a sweep of his hand. This makes them laugh and becomes a game. Still, he will not eat any food. He's agitated from a full day of therapies. We quickly clean up, push him back to his room in the wheelchair, and help him into bed. Gingerly, I unhook his helmet, lift it off and set it on the nightstand. With a kiss, I whisper, "Goodbye Hugh. Have a good night."

He looks at me with his forehead furrowed, "Where are you going?"

"Home," I answer.

"Where's that?" he asks. The girls' eyes widen.

"Our house in Glen Allen, Hugh, the one we bought from Lawrence. Don't you remember it?"

He looks into our faces one by one, thinking hard. The girls and I stand stiff and flabbergasted. Unfazed, he finally shakes his head *no*, sinks back on his pillow and closes his eyes, lapsing into the heavy breathing of sleep within seconds.

The three of us drift through the silent halls and hospital doors, to the elevator and down the ramp; we wind our way around the parking deck, each one of us shaking our heads, each one of us in turn saying out loud and to ourselves, "Oh My God, Dad doesn't know where we live." There's a shock in our voices that trails off into a vaporous silence.

There is another mission to complete before returning home, though, and not much time to process this latest shift in our knowledge of his condition. At Kohl's we buy Hugh several new outfits for rehab. The girls and I stock up on sweats, comfortable shirts, and iron-on labels. I stay up late ironing nametags on all his new things and writing RAWLINS in block letters on the heels of his sneakers.

Weekends at the hospital are rest periods for patients in brain rehab. We all pile on the bed to watch "Fear Factor," a TV show where contestants challenge each other in daring feats and eat disgusting live insects like cockroaches. "That is so gross!" Mary screams. "It's even mean to the cockroaches!" Anna squishes against her father's shoulder, plugging her ears, with one fascinated eye open. Hugh is glued to the physical challenge portion of the show. He pinches Anna's side to startle her and smiles when she screams. I try to imagine we are at home, on the couch, or in the movies—anywhere but here. If I close my eyes and listen to the three of them, it feels that way.

Trudging to the kitchen early Saturday morning, I think: *isn't the weekend supposed to be relaxing?* The flyer on the fridge shouts: Reminder: Shuffles Car Wash. It is May fourth already. I feel crummy, skip the coffee and opt for tea, then drop Anna and Mary at the BP station to raise money for their dance company. Hugh is lying down when I arrive at the hospital and doesn't see me walk in. When I say hello in my raspy bronchitis voice, he doesn't look up. "Nice to meet you," he responds. This is the greeting he offers to all the new nurses, therapists, and aides he meets each day.

"Hugh, it's me, Rosemary." He looks up confused. He has trouble reconciling me with my new voice. "It's me, Hugh. I just have a cold." His nurse asks if we'd like to walk down the hall and he nods. Since there are no therapies today, this will provide a mini workout for him. The nurse walks on one side of him and I walk on the other. Three weeks after the accident we walk down the hall together, holding hands.

"Remember when we used to walk around the block at night like this?" I ask him. He looks at me and nods. But I am learning that there are things he says he remembers that he doesn't. He is not intentionally fibbing; he simply knows he should remember certain things, so he forms the memory at that moment and agrees to believe it to fill in the gap. He also sometimes confuses daydreams with real memories. He might think he has done something when he is only thinking about it intensely. The doctors call this "confabulating." Knowing he will need a rest after the walk, I leave him to check on the girls.

Hugh is wide-awake from a nap, attentive and alert when the three of us arrive back at the hospital in the early evening. He calls Mary "Mary Lou" and Anna "Goose," his old nicknames for them. Delighted, the girls climb onto his bed to snuggle.

The nurse strolls in with her clipboard for a cognitive quiz. "Mr. Rawlins, do you know who these young women are?" she asks in a serious voice.

He looks at her with a wry smile and answers, "No. Who are they?" The girls know he is playing a game, but the nurse has no clue.

She points to Mary and asks in her clinical tone, "Do you know who that is?"

Hugh turns his head to Mary and asks without expression, "Who are you?"

Mary giggles. "I don't know. Who am I?" She is blushing.

Hugh's eyes turn soft, "Mary Katherine," he whispers.

The nurse then asks, "And who's that?" pointing to Anna.

Hugh looks at her goofily and responds, "I don't know, but if you find out, would you please tell me?" We all laugh out loud, as the nurse catches on.

Hugh's dry sense of humor becomes a problem on a different occasion when I receive a phone call at home asking if he has a drinking problem. It seems that whenever he is asked if he'd like a drink, he responds, "Yes, I'll have a J.D. on the rocks." When they say he can't have that, he adds, "Okay, then how about a Jim Beam?" He never smiles when he says these things. I assure them he is not a problem drinker; at least he never was in the past. Inside I hope this is the old Hugh resurfacing.

Early Sunday afternoon, Hugh's parents stop in for a visit. Against the whitewash of the walls, father and son are silhouetted in the afternoon light that shines through the window. They face each other on the bed, mirror images of one another, and even without words, they seem to be communicating. Hugh is a gentle and quiet man like his father; they share the same soft voice and exact posture. His father is patient, slow, and kind as he offers Hugh bites of a sandwich or a glass of water. No small talk necessary.

Later that night, a young resident stops by to see Hugh. He had been in the operating room and is clearly amazed at Hugh's rapid progress. While the doctor is visiting, I ask, "Anyone want a cracker?" and Hugh answers, "Polly." It's an old joke I've heard his parents tell many times. The doctor laughs at his wit, but a little later, when we are alone in the hall, he says something that sticks in my mind and makes my stomach turn over all night. He says he cannot believe how great Hugh is getting along "after seeing his brain pour out like toothpaste in the operating room." Too stunned to respond, I secretly vow to throw out all the pink toothpaste in my house as soon as I get home—only minty green toothpaste from now on.

Chapter 15

Dear Hugh, Rosemary and Family,
It takes great strength, love and belief to get through such a painful and serious
injury. I pray for you with that in mind and have faith that yours will get you
through. Love to each of you as your favorite person takes his time to heal and
joy returns. All our love,
Angela, Larry, and Family

-The McNaughtons, Rosemary's cousins

Days 24-25

"Impulsivity and cognitive deficits are issues for Hugh right now," says the resident-in- charge. My in-laws and I are seated around an oval conference table at our first family meeting with Hugh's treatment team, while he sleeps peacefully after a long day of therapy. A doctor, three therapists, a neuropsychologist, and a social worker ruffle and review stacks of paper that contain individual observations and recommendations. Referring to his chart, the physician tells us that Hugh will remain on IV antibiotics until May 15th. He nods at the speech therapist to his right. She begins at once.

"Hugh is having trouble initiating speech. He has problems with auditory comprehension and processing," she reports. "His attention span is severely impaired, and he engages in confabulation from time to time, which means he fills in gaps in his memory by making things up that he thinks happened. Focusing and maintaining attention are being worked on daily." Looking around the faces at the table, she emphasizes, "Hugh also has no idea how to use his time. He needs lots of structure. He's unable to read or comprehend more than three words in a row. He cannot read a whole paragraph simply because he cannot attend to the task that long." I feel my entire body go rigid as I take this in. To maintain my composure, I avoid eye contact with Hugh's parents.

Turning to psychotherapy, the next doctor discusses Hugh's problems with awareness. "Hugh cannot remember that he's been in an accident and that he's in the hospital. He is unaware of his surroundings and his condition much of the time. However, he is beginning to maintain attention in group counseling sessions when cued to do so." She smiles at this tidbit of positive news.

We progress rapidly down the line, listening to each report. It's the end of the day—Monday—everyone wants to go home to dinner. Moving on to physical therapy, we learn that Hugh initially required twice as much help getting in and out of bed as he does now. He needs assistance to go from sitting to standing, but he's improved. He can walk up and down a flight of twelve stairs at most, but not alone. He can ride a stationary bike for five to ten minutes. His trouble maintaining balance while moving is called dynamic balance impairment.

Between speakers, the room is morosely silent. When I was little I would hold my breath in a tunnel for good luck. In long tunnels, I'd feel shaky. I'd tell myself to look for the light. I feel the same suffocating feeling now, like darkness has swallowed me.

Hugh's occupational therapist is talking about dressing and grooming. "He requires varying degrees of help. His clothing has to be set up and laid out. Putting on socks and shoes is most difficult. He also requires assistance with grooming, tooth-brushing, combing, and shaving. Repeated prompting is necessary for all of these activities," she says.

The recreational therapist notes that Hugh requires twenty-five to fifty percent help to perform recreational and leisure activities.

In short, there is nothing he can initiate or do by himself. Why are we all sitting here smiling politely? I want to double over and sob. I glance at my in-laws and see they're watching my reaction. Then, in a pleasant, sing-song voice, the social worker announces to the group,

"And, we have good news today, a tentative discharge date."

I draw in my breath. "A date already?" I ask.

"Yes," she says, "I just want to say that this is tentative, because it may be a little earlier."

"Wow!" I'm breathing hard.

"The discharge date is the fifteenth."

"Of May?" I ask. Rita's forehead creases.

"Yes."

"That's soon," I say.

"The fifteenth is a week from Wednesday," Rita says. "Nine days from now." Her face flushes with concern. *Dear God!* I think. *I thought he'd be in the hospital for another month at least.*

The social worker tilts her head. "It is possible it could be earlier," she says, "because he's doing so well from a functional point of view." *So well? It doesn't sound that way to me.* "The thing that may hold us to the fifteenth is the IV therapy; however, if we can get that taken care of at home, he is really ready for day rehab."

I am stunned—he's only been on this floor for a week. She discusses our insurance and the two local day rehab programs at Health-South and Sheltering Arms that Hugh could attend several hours each day from home. Then she adds, "The other part of our protocol is what we call a therapeutic leave on the weekend, getting Hugh out of the hospital for a few hours. I want to call and check with the HMO to see if they support an overnight leave or a two-day pass. Then, if they can do the antibiotics at home, he might get out earlier."

I cut her off. "How much earlier? A day? Three days? A week?" No answer. She hunches her shoulders in the wait and see gesture.

My mother-in-law moans, "This is a lot to take in."

"Will he have a wheelchair?" I ask.

"No, he's walking too well to require a wheelchair."

"What about supervision? He has a night sitter in here."

"Yes. Twenty-four hour supervision *will* be needed, at least for the first month, but not by a nurse. It could be anyone in your family—someone to be sure he does not get up, take off his helmet, walk away, fall down the steps..."

"What about the middle of the night when we're trying to sleep?

How does that work?" I ask.

"We recommend a couple of things. You could try a baby monitor. You know, a device that let's you hear what's going on."

"Yes, I know what that is. I have twins," I say, sounding edgy.

"Or you could close your bedroom door and hang a bell on it, so if you're a light sleeper it will alert you that he's up." *Sure,* I think, *that's if he makes it to the door before falling and splitting his head open.* Aloud I say, "Well, actually, I'm taking Ambien right now, so that will be a problem. I'll have to stop taking that, I guess." To this remark, I hear nervous laughter.

Hugh's nurse chimes in, "He's pretty active at night, sleeping only about two hours at a time. So really, some way of knowing when he's awake is safest." Tears pool in my eyes. I blink to hold them back. She continues quietly. "I know it's hard, but things should improve over time. For daytime supervision, a deadbolt and key are recommended for the front door and bells on the doors to be sure he does not go outside unattended." *Bells on the doors? Deadbolt locks?* My head is swimming. I'm still stuck on the words, "He's doing so well." *Am I not on the same page? He doesn't even know he's had an accident.* Nervous energy ricochets off the wall. I shift in my chair. My breathing is shallow, but I manage a weak smile through it all; my proper Catholic upbringing never fails. *Am I really up to all this?*

What about a shower? I ask.

Hugh's O.T. responds. "He has had a few bed baths here, but no shower or shampoo." I'm casually informed that Hugh will not have a shampoo in the hospital. They will not allow him to stand in a shower without his helmet on—it's too dangerous. They tell me that I can wash his hair at home carefully without letting Hugh press on his own head for fear he might push too hard on the soft area. I am to wash it for him very gently. At this I laugh out loud, then check myself. *Too dangerous in the hospital, but recommended at home? How does that make sense? I do not relish the idea of feeling his brain right under his scalp—I'm the medical weenie, remember?*

The doctor reiterates that Hugh might have bouts of agitation when he becomes over-stimulated. "And what do we do to help that?" I ask, the tension now squeaking in my voice.

"Keep a quiet house, with low noise, low visual stimulation, soft voices, low light, a serene atmosphere," he says, as though he's said this many times before.

"This is going to be hard with two teenagers," I mutter under my breath, my demeanor disintegrating. I picture Mary and Anna tap dancing on the kitchen floor.

Rita and Hugh sit rigid, their eyes shifting from sorrow to dread. *Mirrors of my own distress*, I think. I feel totally ill equipped and unqualified to care for Hugh at this stage, but at the same time, I think he will do better at home. I want him home. I also want an entourage of medical assistants to move in with us. Rehab will provide a wheelchair for his trial visits to leave and enter the hospital, but upon his release, I'm assured no wheelchair will be needed, just the gait belt and a constant companion for walking. The constant companion will be me.

"You'll also need a temporary disability tag through the Department of Motor Vehicles for six months. I'll approve that for you at once," the doctor says. All the therapists agree that two trial trips home will precede Hugh's release from the hospital. His first visit will be this coming weekend. Meeting adjourned.

I have *five* days to get my act together.

Hugh's mother says to me on the way out of the meeting room, "Dad and I will pick up the parking tag. Cross that off your list." I mouth a thank-you to her.

"I'll come over at night and sit with him," his father says as we make our way to the elevator. "I want to help—I'd like to…"

"You can't stay up all night, every night," I say. "And besides, he can be a handful. He'll want to go on the stairs."

"What else have I got to do?" he smiles. "I can handle him. He'll listen to me."

"It's not that. I'd rather you were available during the day in case I need back-up. We'll figure something out," I tell him. But the truth is: Hugh is strong, wobbly, and incoherent. I don't want him to pull his father down accidentally.

My anxious mind skips from one worry to the next. I'm even sicker over money after hearing Hugh's assessments. Before leaving the team meeting, I asked the physical therapist about driving. She told me

Hugh would not drive for many months, probably not for a year or more, if ever. I decided on the spot to ditch the Windstar the following day. It will eliminate a car payment and lower my insurance. I'd been considering it for some time anyway. "Hey Dad," I say. "Will you have lunch with Hugh tomorrow? I'm going to sell the Windstar van. It keeps breaking down. You just fixed up Hugh's Explorer, so I'll drive that from now on."

"Sure," he says, perking up. The three of us drive home recounting the meeting and our shock over it. "They sure throw people out of the hospital in a hurry these days," his mother says. A thousand to-do list items flash through my mind.

In my frenzied over-the-top way, I spring into action as soon as I arrive home. Jim and Kevin agree to come right over. Kevin suggests we pull up all the throw rugs, put away any cords, and make sure we don't leave obstacles on the floor. "Try to keep shoes in a closet," he suggests, noting several pairs littering the living room. My new full-time job will be yelling at the girls to put their shoes away, I think. He checks out our shower upstairs; we decide we don't need one downstairs, since Hugh can already climb steps. "A handheld shower upstairs and a shower seat will be helpful," says Kevin. "Handrails in the downstairs bathroom would help too."

In bed at night, my brain won't turn off. I dig in my nightstand for the Ambien bottle. Anxious to rid myself of the van early Tuesday, I clean out all the junk and snack wrappers and vacuum the mats. In my usual hurry, I jump in. As if to spite me, the van engine does not turn over. Jeff Willis has to jump it in the cul-de-sac so I can go sell it. "Don't you ever catch a damn break?" he jokes.

While I am signing papers at the dealership, Hugh's father calls my cell phone. "Hello Roe? I hate to bother you, but I am not at the hospital," he says.

"Why? What's wrong?" I ask.

"I went early to have lunch with Hugh, but he's not there." I stop breathing. "I went to his room and his bed was empty."

"WHAT? What do you…"

"No. No. It's okay." He laughs. "It's a funny story. I go over to the desk and the nurse told me that in the morning exercise session, the therapist mentioned a group was going bowling. She said Hugh perked up and wanted to go."

"Hugh is *bowling*? Did you say *bowling*?"

"Yes, as in bowling ball. It was the first time he acted excited about something, so they let him try. The nurse said a group of them went on a bus to some alley in Mechanicsville. AMF, I think. She said they would have lunch out, so I wanted to tell you not to rush. He's not here!" At this, he laughs again.

When I see Hugh's nurse in the afternoon at the hospital, I hear he managed to bowl with a gait belt and helmet. I can't help but fret that someone from his office might have seen him stumble off the handicap bus, led by a canvas strap, all googly-eyed with that blank look on his face. I want to shelter him from the world until he is his old self again. I want his boss to save his job so he can return when he's better. A voice niggles at the back of my mind: *Will he ever be better?* I hear Hugh's voice inside my head again: *stop worrying about everyone else.* I scold my own ego. *For God's sake, Rosemary, he just had some fun. Give it a rest!*

When I enter Hugh's room, I find him reclining on the bed, hands clasped behind his head, legs stretched out and crossed at the ankles, looking as relaxed as can be. He's wearing navy nylon shorts and a t-shirt bearing the faded stains of a messy lunch.

"So, Hugh, how was the bowling trip?" I ask.

"The what?" he asks, crinkling his nose.

"The bowling trip you went on today."

"I did?" He rolls to his side and begins to doze.

"Never mind," I whisper.

Chapter 16

Diary Note to Hugh
Thursday May 9, 2002

Took Ambien at 11:30 but still can't sleep—it's now after 3 a.m. I had a talk with Mary on the couch. She wants to know if the woman that hit you is sorry. We talked things over, but she was still upset. I suggested she focus on your recovery and not make herself sick. By the time she got to bed, I was wound up and since I couldn't sleep, I called the police officer that was at the scene. I told her I had questions I needed answered—I needed to know if the woman who hit you was concerned at all. She had not contacted us once, and that spoke volumes to me about the kind of person she must be. The officer told me you were probably hit at a force of 65 mph, given the offender's 45-50 mph speed and your 20 mph momentum. She informed me that she had given the woman a reckless driving ticket. The officer was understanding and answered my questions as best she could. I told her how hard it was to carry on with my children torn up over this, your life forever altered, and she—the woman who hit you—basically going about business as usual. All I wanted was some sort of acknowledgement of regret from her, no admission of guilt or legal talk, just an "I'm sorry this happened" sentiment. The officer expressed her own regret and was understanding, but could not give me any insight into this woman. Also, you have a two-day pass to come home and I'm scared to death you'll fall and I won't be able to hold you up. I miss you so much. I wish you could talk to me right now and hold me.

Days 26-29

After a miserable night—to bed at four and up at six—I drive the kids to school. I am drained emotionally, physically and spiritually. My head is throbbing. I want to help Mary cope with her feelings, figure out what Anna is thinking, hear *that* woman say she's sorry, and be with Hugh every second. I want control over my life. I want to know what our future holds. Or do I? The future is a deep black hole too frightening to imagine. If I had a crystal ball right now, I swear, I don't know if I'd look. I call Patty King. "Can you drive me to the hospital? I'm a mess."

"Be right there," she says. Behind the wheel, she sends me several quick sideways glances. "Are you alright, Hon?" Her jeweled sunglasses sparkle in the light.

"Not really. I was up most of the night. I talked to the officer who was at the scene. Mary is totally stressed. Anna is all bottled up. I don't know how to help Hugh or myself much less them right now."

Patty pulls over into a parking lot and stops the car to talk. She is the one person I know who has been through something even more horrific than my experience. Her mother had been brutally attacked and murdered years before, so she possesses a perspective and a finely-tuned spirituality that I desperately need. She understands what is happening on a raw emotional level and is totally in sync with my loss. I feel so grateful for her ability to be open to my pain after having had so much of her own.

"Rosemary, when Mama was killed, I thought I would die too. I thought about her all the time and felt bad about Jon and the kids because I was not there for them. I could not stretch myself that far. It's almost too much to ask of one person."

I cut in. "There's so much I want to do and only so many places I can be at once. The hospital, the kids, all the paperwork – I feel buried alive."

"I know. Believe me, I've been there. You have to give it up to God. Forget the future. Get through today. It's easier said than done. But it has to be done." Her voice is soothing and direct. "I heard about a book called *The Power of Now*. You may want to read it." She explains that the book helps to ground a person in the present. "It also helps with strategies to keep you from dreading the future, you know, anticipatory stress. Lord knows, we could both use that," she laughs.

Once at the hospital, I meet with the physical therapist again for gait belt and wheelchair training for Hugh's trial visit home on the weekend. After lunch, I make phone calls to arrange tours at the two local day rehab facilities—Sheltering Arms and HealthSouth—and once appointments are set, I call the insurance company to clear up some questions.

Thick black clouds eclipse the late afternoon sun and severe storm warnings are announced on television. For the first time, we don't visit the hospital at night. Exhausted and spent, I am not up to driving in dangerous thunderstorms after only two hours sleep. Instead, the girls talk to Hugh on the phone. I am impressed that he even answers the phone when it rings by his bed, and saddened by how far I have lowered the bar of expectations for him.

In spite of the deafening thunder, I sleep soundly and dreamlessly, waking at the break of day, my favorite and most productive time. First call, the nurse's station. All well there. I wake the girls for school. "After today, it's the weekend! C'mon, get out of bed!"

While answering my morning emails, the phone rings. It's Rita. "Betty called and said you are not to buy food for tonight. She and David will buy and prepare dinner at your place at six. Steaks on the grill," she says. I better get moving, I think, lots to do before then. Tonight, at our house, we'll have a small family celebration for Krista's graduation from the Master's program at William & Mary College, and Hugh's father's eightieth birthday. Betty and Dave have flown in from Florida.

"Mom, are you picking us up?" Anna asks on the way to school.

"I can. I'll come straight from the hospital right here. Then we can clean the house before everyone comes." The girls jump out of the Explorer and lug their backpacks across the school lawn.

Upon my arrival at the hospital, I find a wheelchair and hospital pass filled out in Hugh's room. His nurse reminds me, "You'll need to pick up his lunchtime meds at the nurse's station tomorrow before taking him home. Drugs have to be signed out and accounted for."

I accompany Hugh to each of his daytime therapies, and we review home safety measures together.

At the end of this long day, Betty places a tall glass of red wine in my hand, not knowing how nervous I feel about the coming hours. Somehow, in her sensible way, she says all the right things. This preamble to our nuclear family reunion feels just right, low key and relaxed.

Betty wants to see Hugh. She tells me he's been more like a brother than a cousin to her. But I had signed a restricted visitor form at the rehab center, as a few doctors advised, with only six local names on the list including the kids, his parents, and me. Hugh is dead tired after rehab, so I tell her it's really not possible. I feel miserable about it since Hugh and I love Betty dearly. But I keep his impending trip home a secret because I want to see how he reacts before inviting others in.

The morning after, I wake up early. Jim and Kevin drive with me to the hospital to pick up Hugh. Mary and Anna decorate the house with welcome home signs and prepare a special menu to encourage him to eat.

The nurse has been grooming Hugh. He's dressed and shaved, waiting in the wheelchair. "Mr. Rawlins, how wonderful that you're going home today," she says. With an expressionless face, he wheels himself out of the ward and through the MCV lobby. The footrests have long since been removed because he can speed around in the wheelchair, cutting corners with his agile bike-handling skills. "Where are my girls?" he asks.

"They're waiting for you at home," I say. He looks confused. "They're excited to see you," I add, winning a smile.

This is my first time with him outside the hospital since April thirteenth. Only a week ago he asked, "Where is home?" I cannot fathom not knowing where home is. Home is base. It's safety. How can that be lost to him? And why does he not seem upset? It's always me who's frazzled.

In the car, Hugh fidgets with the door handles and locks, but his face, gazing out the window, is set in stone. "Do you recognize anything?" I ask. He doesn't answer; he just holds my hand in his lap and continues to stare outside. Then, unexpectedly he asks, "Kevin, how's your dad?" Kevin is genuinely pleased. He thanks him for asking. His father had been ill before Hugh's accident. A few moments later, Hugh asks, "When is the First Union bike race, Jim?" These bits of history recollected are like valuable heirlooms recovered. I squeeze his hand.

When the car pulls into the driveway, Hugh stares at the house. I don't notice any glimmers of recognition on his face. "We're home," I say. "How does it look to you? The boys have been working hard on it while you were in the hospital."

"Thanks," Hugh says softly to Kevin and Jim. "Looks good." Using the gait belt, I guide Hugh up the three wooden steps of our front porch with Kevin's help. Stepping in the front door, we spot Mary and Anna in the family room. They rush to him calling out, "Hey Dad! Welcome home!" The three of them lock arms in a head-touching hug.

"Let's take a walk," I say. Methodically, we visit every room downstairs. I can see Hugh search his memory for something familiar. Did he expect to see our other house, the one we recently sold? We had lived there for ten years. We've only been in this house eighteen months.

Slowly, I walk behind Hugh on the stairs in case he stumbles, one hand holding the belt, the other one clutching the railing. Kevin encourages me as we go. After climbing the steps, Hugh needs a rest, so we sit down on the edge of our bed. "Sixteen stairs! You already broke your record," I say as Hugh slides into a lying position. "No napping yet," I warn. "There's more to see." As we navigate the second floor, I search Hugh's face for clues. He doesn't give much away—doesn't say he remembers. When Hugh looks rested, Kevin observes me using the gait belt to help him downstairs. "I think you've got the hang of it now," he says. "We'll head out and let you guys visit."

Hugh drifts through a blissful afternoon watching television with his girls curled up on both sides of him. He strokes their hair and glances down at their faces. They snuggle against his shoulder, their arms around his chest laughing at the antics and stunts on "Xena Warrior Princess."

At dinner, the girls fuss over him, refilling his plate until he eats more in one meal than he's eaten during his entire time in the hospital, which isn't really all that much. Eating is slow. He uses his right hand to eat a roast chicken leg and two Kaiser rolls. He even manages a few green beans and potatoes. While Anna clears the dishes, Mary carries a chocolate layer cake over to the table. "Check this out! It's your favorite!" she says. He devours an extra large piece.

"I wish you didn't have to go back tonight, Dad," Anna says helping him clean off the crumbs all over his shirt after dessert.

"Back where?" he asks.

"Nothing," she says, looking uncomfortable. He doesn't ask anything further. After a short rest, Jim returns to help me take Hugh back to his hospital room for the night. He is hesitant to leave.

"You'll be coming back home tomorrow for another full family day," I assure him. I see on his face how much he loves it here, and sense that even if he does not remember this house, he remembers that we are *home* to him. His sweet disposition is a relief to me. The trip has been easier than I anticipated. Patty was right. I need to stop fearing the future and dwell in the present. Each moment will inevitably come as it was meant to be.

Chapter 17

May 13, 2002

Please accept these altar flowers from The Church of the Epiphany on Mother's Day with our love and prayers.

-Church of the Epiphany

Days 30-33

This will be a Mother's Day like no other. I lie wide awake at six a.m., unable to fall back asleep, so I creep down to my office and read family emails between sips of hot coffee. An email from my mother fills me with gratitude and with the reminder that Hugh has given me the greatest gift of all: our two daughters.

I have not attended church in several weeks and have a strong urge to feel its solace and sanctuary. I compose a note to our church friends, dress quickly, and drive to Hermitage Road by myself to deliver it personally. Turning in at the sign, "Church of the Epiphany," I notice the parking lot is empty. The early service let out only minutes ago. Inside, Keith emerges from the sacristy straightening his vestment for the next service. After a warm greeting and hug, I look around at the interior.

This church is much smaller and less ornate than the Catholic church of my youth. I think back on my wedding at St. John's Episcopal Church in Huntington, NY on July 1, 1978. We had decided to marry there for personal reasons after a pre-marital counseling session with a Catholic priest, a decision my parents never criticized. At the time, I didn't fully appreciate how adept my parents were at 'letting go' and allowing all of their children to be individuals without imposing their own personal views on them. "God is God," my mother simply said.

Hugh and I later joined an Episcopal church in Vermont where the girls were baptized, and when we moved again, we joined the Church of the Epiphany in Richmond, where Anna and Mary were confirmed. Epiphany is a small, intimate church, close-knit and informal.

I hand Keith the note to read to the congregation later at the service and he assures me everyone will be glad for the news. He invites me to pray with him and we kneel together in the first pew. Somehow, as the two of us pray aloud in the empty church, I feel a strong sense of peace and belief in the power of God's love to transform Hugh's injury. Even without the presence of the congregation, I feel the pull of their collective spirit, and hear the chorus of their voices as we recite familiar prayers.

Unusually serene, I arrive home and wait with the girls for Jim to arrive. He will help me take Hugh home for his second visit. Jim's been taking a lot of time off from work, so when he arrives I ask him, "Is all this time off okay with your boss?"

"Not really, he's kind of pissed off." Glancing at the expression on my face, he shrugs it off. "Not to worry, Hugh is way more important than my job right now."

At the hospital, a petite, soft-spoken nurse sitter named Evonne greets me. As she fills me in on Hugh's activity during the night, I'm impressed by her conscientiousness. "He had a restless night," she says. "But I kept a close watch on him." If we need a nurse sitter at home, I decide I'll do my best to hire her.

On the car ride home, Hugh keeps pushing the automatic window buttons up and down as if fixated on the motion or sound of the glass. Once home, he wants to spend too much time outside on the back porch where his head sweats under the helmet, making it itch. After Mary and Anna coax him back in, he scratches and squirms until he falls asleep. We decide to let him nap until his parents arrive for our barbeque.

An hour later, Hugh's father mans the grill outside while Hugh stumbles around in a clumsy effort to help out. His mom tries talking about the stock market and subjects he might remember, but he appears dazed and tired. Hugh presents her with a box of candy and a card I bought her for Mother's Day, and though she thanks him, she knows he could not have purchased it. As his parents turn to leave, his mother asks me if I'm sure he is ready to return home yet. "I'm afraid we don't have a choice—he's being discharged," I tell her and she nods, resigned, as she looks over at Hugh asleep on the couch. Her tight hug confirms her confidence in me.

A knock on the door brings relief from the silence the girls have been keeping. Rick has come to help get Hugh back to the hospital. The girls wake their father up with kisses on his cheek. When they tell him it's time to go, he doesn't protest, but looks profoundly sad about leaving. Mary and Anna promise him he will be home for good very soon.

Out in the massive parking lot of MCV, Rick lifts the wheelchair from the car trunk and sets it before Hugh, but Hugh will not sit in it. "I want to walk," he says. The air is stifling. The sun scorches the sidewalk and bakes the long covered walkway up to the hospital. I hold Hugh's gait belt as he lumbers up the long ramp, his right arm gripping the railing, his tired left arm dangling. We trudge along very slowly with Rick pushing the wheelchair right behind Hugh to catch him if he falls. As we approach the incline, I see Rick looks worried that Hugh might topple backward. Hugh begins staggering, but will not get in the chair. Like a marathon runner whose legs have bonked, he drags a few steps, a little further, and gasps for air, but will not give up. Finally, about three quarters of the way up, he relents and lowers himself into the seat. When we arrive at his room, he cannot get into bed fast enough.

"Goodbye, Hugh, have a good long sleep now," I say to him, pulling the blanket up under his chin—the air conditioning makes the room feel frigid after the humid outside air. "Thank you for a wonderful Mother's day and for giving me two beautiful babies," I say to him.

His eyes are closed, but he manages a slight smile when he whispers, "You're welcome," then drifts instantly to sleep.

Rick drives home, clearly relieved to have Hugh back safely in his room. "Can you believe the way he walked up that ramp?" he marvels.

"Yes, I can believe it. He has an iron will—stubborn as a mule."

"That's what's getting him through this," Rick says. As we pull up to my house, I step out of Rick's car. "Thanks, I couldn't have done this without you today," I say as I wave goodbye, and walk through my front door.

"Surprise!" Anna and Mary yell. They are each holding a bundle of baby roses for me. I have an instant flashback to a Mother's day long, long ago when their chubby two-year-old hands each gripped a floppy fresh-picked bundle of wild flowers for me.

Mary steps forward and says, "Mom, let's go to Dairy Queen. We'll treat you."

"Yeah, we want you to have some fun on Mother's Day," says Anna. Although every bone in my body wants to flop on the bed, I can't resist their enthusiasm. We drive to Innsbrook where there is a new shopping center. Surrounding the small gift shops and stores are beautifully tended flowerbeds, ponds stocked with fish under short arching bridges, and winding walkways. Feeling lighthearted, we choose our ice cream sundaes and toppings. As we stroll around casually talking between delectable bites, we start seeing people we know. Instinctively we duck them. None of us wants to hear, "How is Hugh? We're so sorry..." We just want to be out together, away from our lives for one hour. We are all on the same wavelength, turning corners when we see familiar faces, until finally we decide to leave.

Disappointed at the way circumstances have put the brakes on our escape, Anna and Mary apologize that it was a rotten Mother's Day. I try to explain to them that being their mother is the highlight of my life, but these words don't convince them. They wanted the day to be special and me to be happy, and they feel like nothing they did could bring a true smile to my face. I fall into bed feeling inadequate in every way and vow to myself that I'll be more upbeat. I reach for the peace I found this morning in church—that feeling of inner quiet and connection, but my mind keeps returning to the disappointment on their earnest faces. I finally reach for the little white sleeping pill that blacks out the chatter in my brain and fall into the welcoming arms of darkness.

Hugh will be home in two days and the house is not ready. There are tripping traps everywhere. Debbie and Patty help me roll up rugs and store them in the attic, put stray shoes away, and check electrical cords that are near walking areas. We inspect the whole house for areas where Hugh might trip, fall, or knock things over. Breakables are stored in closets. The Jack Daniels is hidden as a precaution, and the furniture is better arranged for wide walkways. "Lookin' good. This place is immaculate!" Patty says, washing her hands in the sink.

At the La-Z-Boy store, Jim tries the chair Debbie has chosen for Hugh and tests several others for comparison. He likes the one she has chosen, so we buy it that night—it's a large Hunter green soft weave that boasts several reclining positions with one that is almost flat for sleeping. We lug it home and the girls eagerly rearrange furniture to make it fit in a corner of the family room. Our worn out old loveseat is put in the garage. Jeff Willis quietly comes by, picks it up and takes it to the dump for me the very next day.

Hugh has spent a total of thirty-three days in the hospital. On his last full day there, a final field trip is scheduled with rehab before going home. The recreational therapist takes him, along with others, to Virginia Center Commons mall for burgers and fries at lunchtime. I am glad he is busy because I have to tour two rehab facilities in one day and decide which one he will attend as early as next week. I decide to check out Sheltering Arms first. It's farther from our home. I like the facility. It's new, clean and appears to have a well-qualified staff. There is one major drawback however: distance. It is forty-five minutes from our house each way and Hugh is at high risk for car sickness.

In the afternoon, I visit HealthSouth. It's closer to home, larger inside, and has a new outdoor movement center where people learn to walk on different surfaces: gravel, grass, cement, stairs, and ramps. This will improve his balance. There is a pleasant alfresco eating area as well, and the staff appears competent and helpful. I choose HealthSouth.

Arriving home just in time to meet the girls, I realize that a month has passed and I have not once resumed my old life—no work, no social life. Every minute revolves totally around Hugh's recovery. I wonder what people do who don't have any insurance or have to go to work every day. I suspect they lose their jobs or have to entrust their loved ones to someone else's care at great expense. At least we are getting by.

On his last night in the hospital, Hugh shares a pizza with the girls. As they all crowd on the bed eating, I am folding up clothes to take home. A young resident walks in holding a clipboard for a final cognitive assessment and memory study.

"Mr. Rawlins, if you don't mind, could you answer a few questions for me?" Hugh nods yes. Everyone stops chewing for a minute.

"Do you remember anything about the accident?"

"No."

"Do you remember anything before the accident—where you were, what you might have been doing?"

"No."

"What is the last thing you remember before the accident?"

"I don't know."

"Where are you now, Mr. Rawlins?"

Hugh looks around the room thoughtfully. He's sitting on a cranked bed with an IV in his hand. The resident is wearing a white coat with a nametag. A sliding curtain is pulled to one side revealing a waste can with the marking: "Infectious Material Only."

The resident repeats, "Mr. Rawlins, can you tell me where you are now?"

"In a government building?" he guesses.

I cannot believe my ears.

Chapter 18

"Great news, Roe. We are all so glad he is making it through. I'm sure he will beat all speed records for recovery. And he gets to fall in love with you all over again — what a lucky guy!
John

        -My brother, in response to a note that Hugh has lost some memory

Discharged from Hospital: May 15, 2002
Day 33

The girls are up early and excited today. They have the day off from school and their dad is coming home to stay. Mary wraps up the newly crocheted blanket she and Anna have finished for Hugh. Jim is standing by the kitchen table shaking his head in amazement at the amount of food Anna can stuff down for breakfast: several pieces of French toast, a sliced apple with cinnamon and sugar, and a whole English muffin, all washed down with two large glasses of orange juice. "Where do you put all that food, Anna? You look like you don't even weigh a hundred pounds," he laughs. Jim has offered to drive for us so I can help Hugh in the car if he becomes agitated.

"You've taken a ton of time off from work on our account. Sure it's okay?" I ask again.

"Not really, but I'm doing it anyway," he says.

"You remind me of Hugh when you talk like that. Don't get fired because of us."

"You have bigger things to worry about than me. Don't even think about it." When my eyes tear up he says, "Let's get going, that is, if Anna's done eating!"

We stop by the ICU and deliver a few thank you cards before entering the Brain Rehab Unit. Hugh is sitting up in bed with a broad smile on his face when we peek in. He knows he is coming home for good. We pack up his room and photograph Hugh with each of his therapists. Before leaving, he needs his discharge papers, but they're not ready yet.

For fun, Hugh pushes Anna in the wheelchair. Her legs fly up when he surprises her with a strong push and she lets out a scream as he sends her flying down the hall. "Dad, slow down!" Everyone is in a good mood, anxious to get Hugh out of the hospital. We wind up in the family room seated together on the large couch blowing up rubber surgical gloves into balloons to amuse ourselves. As the girls sit on either side of their father, Hugh blows up his white rubber glove. Slowly and deliberately, he folds down all the fingers but the middle one. The girls giggle, "DAD!" which only makes him more determined to make them laugh again. Glancing over at the back of his wheelchair, he reads the brand name aloud: "Quickie," and begins grabbing for me. "Hey Roe, how about a quickie?" The girls roll their eyes and choke with repressed laughter.

"C'mon, Hugh, that's enough," I say, checking my watch again and looking toward the door for the doctor.

Jim walks the girls down to McDonald's to pick up burgers at lunchtime. After eating, we throw balled-up wrappers in the wastebasket to kill time. At last, a rehab doctor stops by, chart in hand. He says to Hugh, "Remember, when you get home, listen to the boss," and he points in my direction.

Hugh replies, "The last time I didn't, she smacked me upside the head and that's why I'm here!" I just shake my head - a short while ago he didn't even know he was in a hospital.

"Okay. You're done. Take care," smiles the doctor as he signs the release form.

Once home, Hugh's parents join us. The girls and I prepare a complete out-of-season Thanksgiving dinner with turkey and all the trimmings. Hugh eats heartily and settles into his new recliner for a nap, a look of pure contentment on his face. In the evening, Kelly picks the girls up and takes them to dance. While I have Hugh alone in the house, I decide it's time to get him in the shower. He has not had a real bath in thirty-three days.

Using my gait belt skills, I guide him up the stairs. Once in our bedroom, he needs a rest before we can venture into the shower stall nearby. Our shower has a corner seat, but it's a bit small. I help him wash his head very gently and scrub him thoroughly, carefully monitoring his balance. Once he's wrapped in a towel, I ask him how much he thinks he weighs.

"195" he answers firmly. He was 198 pounds when he was admitted to the hospital.

"I'd be surprised if you weigh 170. You are skinny as a rail."

"No way!" He makes me a five-dollar bet that he weighs 195, give or take a pound. When he stands on the scale, it reads 160. Hugh has lost over a month of memory. For him, the calendar stopped flipping around the time of the accident. I don't know how he explains the weight loss to himself or what he is thinking. He only says, "Let's talk about it later," as if it doesn't matter. I put a hot pack on his back and he slides into a nap. I can't help but think—wouldn't this be every woman's dream—to wake up and be thirty-eight pounds thinner without even knowing how she did it! After dance, the girls run upstairs and jump onto our bed, jolting Hugh awake.

"Hey, careful," I say. Hugh just smiles. The girls delight him with stories from the jazz studio. His groggy eyes crease with delight.

"Girls, Evonne's coming over at ten, and I'm going right to bed, so I can let her out at six in the morning—just letting you know, this is my new bedtime," I say. On the fly, I purchased a wingback chair at a furniture warehouse earlier in the week. The entire unplanned shopping excursion took exactly fifteen minutes. Now the chair sits near the bed in the guest room where Hugh will sleep.

At ten sharp, Evonne arrives. I run down and greet her while the girls wait with Hugh in our room. When I say, "Hugh, it's Evonne from the hospital," he acts pleased to see her, although I can tell he has no idea who she is. After we say goodnight, I ask Evonne if she wants any water, snacks, or magazines. In her serious tone, she says, "No, thank you. I'm not taking my eyes off him!"

After reading a little and saying goodnight to everyone, I set my alarm for five forty-five so I can hear a report about Hugh's nighttime activity before taking over for the day. All of us feel comfortable with Evonne in the house and relieved to have her help. She's not intrusive and her presence is reassuring. Hugh keeps her busy with his midnight jaunts downstairs for chocolate teddy grahams, trips to the bathroom, and walks around the house with no destination in mind. He is a nocturnal creature, active and restless in the dark, with a body that shuts down in the early morning hours. His frequent daytime naps contribute to his daytime sleepiness, but they are absolutely essential to his healing brain.

Trying to get Hugh out of bed in the morning is like trying to pull a hibernating bear from its den. He will not budge. With eyes closed, he grumbles, "Five more minutes." Then he sleeps another ten minutes. I wake him, and we start the cycle again. His resistance requires more strategic tactics: I pull the covers off him.

"Hey, you're mean. It's cold!" he complains.

"I've already woken you up three times. Give me a break," I protest. Finally, he trudges to the bathroom with slumped shoulders and a defiant chin. I help him brush his teeth by saying the steps as I was instructed in the hospital. "First put the toothpaste on the brush. Okay, now it's time to shave." He does not like shaving and has started to grow a goatee.

"Hugh, can you please shave?" I plead, standing in the doorway, blocking his exit.

"I did already," he says.

"I've been standing her the whole time. You have not shaved."

"I'm growing a mustache, a Fu Manchu."

"Why now?"

"I always had one," he says, as if I'm stupid.

"You have not had a mustache in years, Hugh." He raises his eyebrows as if to say, "Wanna bet?" The conversation is over. Hugh will not shave again this morning and now he won't talk to me either. He pushes past me to go downstairs and gives me a look that says, "You can let go of my gait belt now." He looks grungy and neglected, but there's little I can do about it, so I decide to forget it and pick my battles. I'm in no shape for battle anyway.

Not a single day wasted, we meet Dr. Giordano the day after Hugh arrives home, on the morning of May 16th. Dr. G, as he's commonly known, conducts a full round of assessments to set up a team of therapists for Hugh in the Day Rehab Program at HealthSouth. The doctor asks Hugh to count backwards by sevens from 100, and he does so fairly easily. The doctor then gives him a few word memory tests and says his post-traumatic amnesia is beginning to clear. A "smell" test determines that Hugh has lost his sense of smell, which the doctor says contributes to his not wanting to eat. "It may or may not return," he says. Hugh's eyesight cannot be tested now, since the results would be inconclusive because the brain has not yet healed enough. Problems with attention, concentration, balance, and reasoning, as well as other cognitive deficits will be evaluated by the speech therapist.

Dr. G asks Hugh, "Do you know why you need treatment?"

Hugh responds, "I was hit by a car." For the first time, he answers this question correctly, yet it blows my mind that he states it blandly, as if he had memorized it for a quiz. He's not alarmed that he has been severely injured and requires months of rehabilitation. I cannot understand this! I want to see a reaction!

Dr. G determines that Hugh has significant loss of function on his left side, which is a problem since Hugh is left handed, but the doctor feels Hugh's speech is good. He predicts a steady recovery since all of his prognosticators are strong. Some of the indicators of how a TBI patient will fare include: age, intelligence and level of education, history of drug or alcohol abuse, supportive family, supportive friends, and general health prior to the injury. All of his indicators are positive.

"It is common for TBI patients to have periods of recovery followed by plateaus," the doctor says. "The therapists will continually test Hugh to see that he is challenged and moving forward, but if he begins to plateau, therapy may stop for awhile until he begins to show improvement again." In short, the insurance company does not want to pay for therapy that doesn't get results. As long as Hugh continues to improve, he will continue therapy. During a plateau, therapy will be suspended for a period of time. Once he reaches his final plateau, and there are no further significant gains from therapy, his visits will stop altogether, and from that point on we will begin our post- injury life in whatever state he's in. There are no promises about what that end condition might look like. It is unknown, but expectations are that some significant improvements will be made.

The doctor then presents us with two sobering statistics. He states that many couples divorce in the first few years following a severe traumatic brain injury, and a large percentage experience financial distress. The doctor also warns us that Hugh might become verbally abusive or act out due to his injury and we should both be mindful of it and try to keep things under control together. "I'm not trying to scare you. I just want you to be aware of this and to try to be considerate of each other, be tolerant, and plan for the future as best you can," he counsels. We both appreciate his frankness and I really appreciate the way he interacts with Hugh. He gives his undivided attention to him, and takes great care to understand and allow Hugh to clarify his feelings.

Next, we meet the nurse. She takes Hugh's medical history and gives him a pen to sign his name. Hugh's weak grip causes the pen to keep slipping out of his left hand before he can make a single mark. He stares at the paper, then at the pen in fierce concentration, but cannot get a single stroke on the page. She is patient, coaxing him gently with good humor; she tells stories about her kids to break the tension and gives him time to concentrate. Finally, after what seems like hours, she quietly puts her hand on the pen and waits for Hugh's eyes to meet hers. "You can try again tomorrow, Hugh," she says. This is my first lesson in rehab. Never say, "Forget it." Always say, "Try again later."

At home, dinnertime is awkward. The family sits around the kitchen table for a dinner of baked ziti, salad, and warm garlic bread, heavy on the garlic, to entice Hugh to eat. We watch as he painstakingly lifts his left hand, slowly reaches for his fork, and picks it up. The fork dangles like a wind chime as he raises it. It looks like a magic trick, like he's raising the fork without actually touching it. We stare at him, hypnotized. He has blocked out the scene around him as he uses all his concentration to *will* the fork to his mouth to eat, only he can't make it work. It is hard to know what to say. The girls sweetly encourage, "It's alright, Dad, use your other hand." He will not look up at them or acknowledge the remark. Finally, he gives up. "I'm not hungry at all," he says, retreating to his recliner. Mary helps him with the gait belt to walk the few steps to his chair and settle in. He stares ahead in a sorrowful daze. Anna and I clear the dishes away in silence. We have all lost our appetites.

At HealthSouth in rehab, his PT and OT work with him to strengthen his left hand. He practices grasping different sized pegs and inserts them into a drilled-out board. He is introduced to a thick foam gripper that he can put a number of things inside to help pick things up: a pen, a fork, or toothbrush. This allows him to practice grasping with his left hand, which will improve his fine motor skills. Even with the gripper, grasping with his left hand proves nearly impossible for him at first. If he gets too frustrated, he's instructed to use his right hand to do the things he needs to do, but the therapist stresses he should use his left hand whenever possible. Using his right hand is considered a "compensatory strategy," a substitute for his regular habits, to be used as a last resort.

Early one morning, Evonne decides to stay a little later to help me get Hugh out of bed. We figure someone other than a wife may be more successful at getting him up and going.

"Mr. Rawlins," she says in her professional voice, "it's time to get up out of bed."

"No thank you," he answers politely while pulling the covers over his head. We look at each other, stifling a laugh. At last, Mary comes in and promises him a hug if he meets her downstairs while she eats breakfast. This gets him out of bed. Before going downstairs, we talk him into shaving. Evonne is in the doorway and I am in the bathroom standing next to him as he looks in the mirror and begins to shave with the electric razor. Suddenly he collapses, but Evonne and I catch him. He falls into a dead weight and the two of us drag him onto the bed just a few feet away. He's awake. "Hugh, what happened?" I ask.

"I don't know. I just got woozy."

After his color returns, Evonne helps me guide him downstairs, where he spends five minutes with the girls before they leave. It's time for Evonne to go home, so I let her out while he's talking to the girls over toast. For these first few days of rehab, I am his driver. Suddenly, this feels like more than I can handle alone. I'm afraid he'll have another dizzy spell on his way out to the car and I won't be so lucky this time.

Ed and Margaret Martin had told me they were home most of the time in case I need help. I call and they come over almost immediately. Ed brings a surfing magazine and video for Hugh and drives us to HealthSouth in our Explorer. Margaret follows us to drive Ed home. I stay at HealthSouth with Hugh so I can see his routine there.

In the afternoon, Margaret returns. She comes inside to help me get Hugh into the car and meets me in the "day room," a room full of comfortable rocking chairs and leather recliners with a TV and magazines where patients wait between therapies or rest at the end of the day. Margaret and I find Hugh folded into a comfy chair sound asleep, and gently wake him up. His eyes fly open, wild and startled. We help him steady himself and rise out of the chair. He is so tired from his day of therapy that he can barely walk the short distance to the car parked directly outside.

As we pull into the driveway, I see our dentist, Dr. Norris, mowing our lawn! He waves at us happily. "Just about finished," he hollers. I help Hugh over the threshold and into his soft green recliner and carefully remove his helmet. As I unclasp it, Dr. Norris knocks once, before walking in from the garage to the kitchen. Hugh asks the doctor, "How do you like my brain bucket?"

An amused smile glints in the doctor's eyes. "It's pretty neat. How are you feeling these days, Hugh?" Dr. Norris heads to the kitchen sink to wash up. The summer is unusually dry and he's covered in a fine film of dust kicked up by the mower. He scrubs both hands and forearms in his meticulous medical way, then splashes his face and turns to hear Hugh's reply, while dabbing his face with a dishtowel.

"I'm fine. Thanks for mowing the lawn," Hugh says.

"Hey, it's my pleasure. I get to ride on the tractor. I love it!"

Dr. Norris chats a little as Hugh rises up out of his chair and walks him to the foyer with me. I'm holding onto Hugh's belt since his helmet is off. "How are your teeth, Hugh? Has anyone checked your mouth since the accident?"

Hugh looks at me, eyebrows furrowed. He doesn't know the answer to that question. I explain to Dr. Norris that Hugh is not allowed any Novocain yet, so we have put it off for the time being. We promise to have his teeth checked after his bone flap operation.

"Mind if I have a look?" the doctor asks, stretching up toward Hugh.

Hugh stands in the foyer, mouth wide open, as Dr. Norris peeks in.

"Hmm, chipped front tooth, maybe a cavity or two. Nothing we can't wait to deal with though. You got off easy, considering."

Once Dr. Norris leaves, Hugh pushes back into his recliner with a wide yawn. Settling in with a dreamy look of satisfaction, he says proudly, "I bet I'm the only guy whose dentist will mow his lawn." It is clear he is touched and flattered by the kindness as he pulls his blue crocheted blanket up, contentedly hooking the corners over his shoulders. His head flops to one side, and in an instant, he's asleep, the slanted half smile still on his face.

Usually, Hugh sleeps for a few hours after rehab. This is precious time for me to make phone calls. I have found out that our insurance company will not cover the night sitter. They view it as custodial care rather than required medical care. I find it upsetting but mildly amusing that the sitter was "required" in a hospital full of medically trained doctors and nurses in order to keep Hugh from being tied to the bed, yet a sitter is not necessary in a house with a wife and two teenagers who have no medical training whatsoever. I decide to see if I can do something about it while I pay Evonne out of my savings account, watching it deplete at an alarming rate. I write letters, make inquiry calls, and have doctors write notes of recommendation to no avail. I still have to pay out of pocket to the tune of several hundred dollars a week. Evonne and the peace of mind she affords us are worth every penny.

I have decided that each weekend Evonne will take Saturday night off, so I can see if I can get through the night with Hugh alone. This first Saturday afternoon with Hugh home, Kevin and Jim come over for a few hours. Kevin shows Hugh some exercises for his arm. The girls and I take off shopping in a giddy mood. Mary shows me her artwork on exhibit in the atrium of the Virginia Center Commons Mall, and I take pictures of her painting to share with Hugh. The girls and I spend a lighthearted afternoon window shopping and checking out the latest fashions with a side trip to Chick-Fil-A for three orders of waffle fries.

On Saturday night, Hugh and I return to our own bed together for the first time. Climbing into the covers next to him fills me with a wave of affection and remembrance of things I have not thought about in years: our first kiss, our most intimate moments. I am thankful he is alive and cannot believe he is next to me. Slowly, he turns toward me in the dark. He's lying on his right side. His left arm is weak but it rises in the air between us and settles on my face. His fingers tremble over me silkily, across my cheek, down my neck, and onto my breast. He inches closer before his hand settles heavily on my waist, exhausted by the effort. Thinking he's asleep, I stir a little. His arm tightens around me. He is awake and begins exploring. I am more than a little surprised at what he wants.

Our coming together is so much more than physical. There is an urgency we need to express to each other, a depth of emotion that is almost painful. Hugh moves in slow motion as he holds my hips. The tender, light touch of his left hand is excruciatingly erotic, and his right hand is strong. He drags his left arm across my body, brushing my skin with his weak fingers. At intervals, he lets his heavy hand rest, and pauses with eyes closed, breathing on my skin. Just when I begin to doze off, he caresses me again. We hug for long quiet periods and I move under him as tears pour down my face. Hugh's short-term memory lapses cause him to caress me again and again with no recollection that we had made love an hour ago. He slowly devours me, dozes off, and then embraces me again as if it's the first time.

I remember the desperate lovemaking of our youth and the interludes we had as young parents—always tired, with little privacy—always rushed. As the girls grew older, our intimacy took on a familiarity, a pattern. Romance was scheduled and predictable. But this night is a gift of yearning and fulfillment. In the darkness, I can envision Hugh as he was before, strong and commanding, yet gentle. Every second is sacred, the active and the passive. In the final moments before morning, I sob openly as he holds me. Hugh whispers, "Thank you," then falls into a deep sleep just before dawn. An hour later, he stirs.

"You awake?" I whisper.

"Uh-huh," he says.

"What an amazing night. You were so loving…"

"What? What'd we do?" he asks. Every cell in my body freezes. "What? Tell me," he says in a louder voice, seeing my reaction. I rise from the bed feeling cheated.

"Nothing. Forget it," I say, "I'll get you some tea. Stay in bed." I run from the room, down the stairs to the kitchen; I slam a teacup on the counter and nearly break it. *Why God? Why?* My entire body vibrates with unreleased grief.

My husband and I can reminisce about our wedding and the birth of our twin daughters together, but he will never remember two of the most defining nights of my life with him. The first, and most frightening, the night he almost died. The other, the most passionate, intense night of lovemaking we have ever shared. These events are wiped from his memory forever. Even though I am locked into both turning points with him, I am alone in my recollections. They shape my emotional future, but have little impact on his. I have never felt more alone.

I walk a wide circle in the kitchen, breathing wildly, wanting to hit something. I smash both fists on the kitchen counter, lay my head on my forearms, and cry. *But he did it. He loved me. It was real. He made me believe we could …* unexpectedly, I smile at the solid memory of his touch. There is still a strong physical connection between us, a loving bond that is tighter than ever. I know if Hugh can be with me this intimately, this contentedly so soon after his accident, we still have many good memories to make. For the first time since the accident, I imagine a future with him, not just as a caregiver, but also as a partner and a lover.

He's sitting up when I reenter the bedroom with a tray. "Blueberry muffin. Yum!" he says, looking up at me. I kiss him hard on the mouth.

"What was that for?" he asks.

"For last night," I say.

Chapter 19

Five to six weeks out

Hugh drifts back asleep after his muffin. While lying next to him, too tired to read the newspaper, I doze off for what feels like a minute, then suddenly my eyes fly open to see him falling backward with no helmet on his head. I leap off the side and catch him just in time, dragging him back onto the mattress.

"What happened?" I ask.

"It feels like I was tackled from behind."

"I was catching you, not tackling you. Are you dizzy?"

"I guess," he says. You should be, I think, you were certainly busy all night! For the next hour, I lie awake, not daring to sleep in case he gets up again and falls. Once he's in a deep sleep, I sneak away for the phone and call Evonne to tell her we'll need her again this week.

Now that I'm familiar with Hugh's routine at HealthSouth, he'll be going alone. Our insurance covers the expense of a door-to-door taxi with trained drivers to guide him to the car and drive him to rehab. I'm relieved I don't have to do it by myself. Knowing Hugh has trouble waking up, I rouse him early, so we can begin the slow process of grooming and dressing, and still have time for breakfast before the driver arrives. Cheerful at first, my mood changes after he falls back asleep twice.

"Hugh, this is the third time I've woken you up. It's getting late. You need to get up."

"Who says so?" he demands. "Why do you always have to have things *your* way?" He pulls the covers over his head.

"The cab's due in fifteen minutes. The therapists at HealthSouth are waiting for you. Please get up."

"I'll get up later," he grunts, glaring at me before slowly rolling over. I pull the quilt off him. He cuts his eyes at me, stumbles out of the bed and into the bathroom, pulls a large towel from the rack, and trips back to bed. As he curls up in his terry cloth blanket, I take five deep breaths to control my anger.

"This towel isn't warm anyway," he rumbles as he tries to sit up, his way of giving in. I lay his clothing out for him. He focuses and concentrates on each piece to put the right garment on in the correct order. He does most of it nearly one-handed, which drags the process out longer. Fighting down the urge to help him takes practice. We are living life in extreme slow motion, a nerve-fraying pace for someone like me.

Once he leaves for rehab, I call the doctor about Hugh's difficulty staying alert. He suggests we stop Hugh's sleeping medicine on a trial basis, since it may be making him too groggy during the day.

Later, when Hugh is wide-awake, we talk. "Why do you give me such a hard time in the morning?" I ask.

"I know I'm hard on you. I can't explain it," he laments, "I'm just so tired, not the normal tired, an impossible tired. It's like my body is a cement block. I can't think straight. I promise I'll get up on time tomorrow."

"You always promise, then you don't. I hate that you get mad at me for waking you up."

"How about I write you a note promising to get up. I'll sign it right now. Then I'll believe you when you say I promised." I print up an agreement on the computer, a silly two-liner, and he signs the bottom with his messy right-handed scrawl, "Your deviant, Hugh." I place the note on his nightstand.

Kelly drives the girls to dance and Peggy T. drops them home. With all my friends taxiing Mary and Anna, I hardly see them lately. They burst in the door at 9:30 full of energy. Thirty minutes later, Evonne arrives for the night.

"We're going to try skipping the sleeping pill tonight," I tell her.

"Good thing I rested a bit today," she says smiling. Once everyone settles in, I swallow my Ambien and slip into bed.

In the morning, Evonne reports that Hugh did not fall asleep until two a.m. after they made a trip downstairs for a midnight snack. Then he slept fitfully. He needs to be woken up by seven for rehab. I talk to the girls and we decide to try tenderness. Anna prepares a breakfast tray of tea, English muffins, and cantaloupe. Mary sits on the bed next to him, rubbing his shoulder. "C'mon Dad, try to eat something, and let's get ready. You're lucky! You get to go to the gym all day. I have to go to math," she says, nudging him, but he's sluggish. The girls have to leave for school before he's done eating, so they kiss his cheek and run down the stairs with backpacks. In the short time it takes me to see them to the front door and wave them off, Hugh has fallen back to sleep. As I shake his shoulder to wake him, he says groggily, "Don't forget to send the girls in for a kiss before school."

"They kissed you goodbye two minutes ago, honey. They're gone."

"Oh. Where'd they go?" He looks at his cold English muffin.

"To school," I say, exasperated.

He looks perplexed. I show him the note we had prepared the day before about getting up in the morning. He points to the word deviant. "I wrote that?" he asks.

"Yes, you did," I say.

"Oh, yeah, now I remember." He's pleased with himself. "Okay, but I'm not shaving!" he says. "And these sweat pants are fine. I don't need to change." *Yuck*, I think, but I don't argue. I'm getting used to his new look. What shall we call it: the midlife grunge or the deviant debonair?

After rehab, Hugh is obviously overtired. He bolts for the recliner—in his newfound bolting way, which isn't really a bolt, but a slow, desperate attempt to rush to the chair. He grabs the remote off the end table and dismantles it completely while complaining that it doesn't work. Between pressing the remote buttons over and over again, he dozes on and off. His parents stop by for a short visit before driving the girls to hip-hop. Jim also stops by to chat since he was passing our house on his bike ride. "It's not a great time, Jim," I say, without inviting him in. After he leaves, I feel like a lousy friend, but I'm too cranky and miserable to be civil.

When Hugh wakes up, I tell him it's time for dinner. He's bleary-eyed and tells me he only loves me a little because I'm a nag and I do everything fast. He delivers this news in a monotone. I want to yell, "I don't love you so much right now either," but I know it's not true and immediately strike the words from my thoughts when he tells me his head hurts, it itches, and he wishes he could just sleep forever.

Eventually, I cajole him into the shower and wash his scalp with dandruff shampoo as recommended by Dr. Ward. Crusted over with scabs and dry, flaky skin, his head itches so furiously that he sometimes scratches it until it bleeds. While I'm at it, I scrub the dried blood from his fingernails too. Afterward, we both collapse on the bed to vegetate.

As we adapt to our new schedule this week, we both feel out of sorts. Hugh attends rehab by himself and I have a few hours alone at home, but find myself thinking about him all the time. I'm told that Hugh sleeps through frequent breaks at rehab as they work with him on his orientation of time and place. He arrives home early in the afternoon completely exhausted and sleeps in his recliner. This new schedule allows me to tend to chores that have been neglected over the past several weeks, so I collect my energy and try to get back to work.

Returning to my résumé writing business is a gift I present to myself. I have been out of work for over a month. As I sit in my office with Hugh, right inside the front door, the doorbell rings.

"Ready Mr. Rawlins?" asks the taxi driver as he takes firm hold of Hugh's gait belt. Hugh kisses me in the foyer and leaves the house dressed for a cold fall day in sweats, which would be fine, except that it's May in Virginia. Even though it's nearly eighty degrees, he feels cold all the time. I'm told it's one of the quirky symptoms of TBI. Hugh is so cold; he never wants to get into the shower because that feels *really* cold. I warm up his towels in the dryer to coax him, but then he bundles up contentedly for an hour or more, not wanting to take the warmed towels off to dress.

I'm checking the calendar to review my schedule when the phone rings. "Résumés Worth Reading, Rosemary Rawlins speaking," I answer.

"Hi Hon." It's Hugh.

"Where are you?" I ask. *Has he escaped rehab? Is he wandering the streets?*

"I'm in the day room waiting for my next appointment," he says casually. "I'm on the courtesy phone." I smile because he initiated the phone call. I can't help but feel a sense of accomplishment for him.

"Are you okay?" I ask.

"Yeah. I was just thinking about you and thought I'd call. I have a headache, though. Can you get me some something for it when I get home?"

Instead of suggesting that he's in a healthcare facility where they have pain pills, I just say, "Sure." It feels good to finally solve a problem. While we chat, it's fun to imagine he's calling me from work like the old days. I call Dr. Ward about the headache and he says they're common and will probably continue for a while. The phone call from Hugh is a complete surprise. I find out later, he made other calls too. I speak to Michelle, his administrative assistant, that afternoon.

"Omigod! Rosemary, Hugh called me at the office. At first I wasn't sure it was him, I was so surprised."

"Really?"

"Yeah, he told me he was bouncing a ball in rehab. He said he missed work. It was so great to hear him on the phone."

"I'm so glad, Michelle. I think he's feeling better. We'll see you later." I silently wonder how many people he's called and what on earth he is saying to them. Bouncing a ball? How is that going over at the office? On the other hand, I'm relieved to see he has remembered all of his old office phone numbers.

Early evening, Michelle arrives with extra spicy chicken wings for dinner while the girls are at dance. Hugh still has no sense of smell and requests everything with piles of red pepper on it. Michelle tells Hugh about some changes that are going on at the office and reminds him that everyone misses him. After she leaves, I guide Hugh upstairs to the back room to watch T.V. When Evonne arrives, we find Hugh sitting on the bed, strapping on his gait belt and helmet. It's nearly ten p.m. "Where are you going, Mr. Rawlins?" she asks in her calm way.

"Hi Evonne. It's good to see you," he says.

"It's good to see you too. But you still didn't answer my question. Are you going somewhere?"

"Just down the hall to see my daughters." She crosses the room with her arms out.

"Here, let me help you with that." Because of his left hand weakness, Hugh has trouble buckling his helmet. Evonne secures it to his head. They walk down the hall together and knock on Mary's door. "Who is it?" Mary calls out.

"A secret admirer," her dad answers.

The door swings open. "Daddy!" shouts Mary, "You came to visit me!" They sit on the bed and talk, holding hands.

After a while, he says, "Now I need to go see Goose. Where is she?"

"She's in her room, Dad." He kisses Mary on the cheek and they say good night.

Evonne escorts him down the narrow hall to Anna's room. He sits on Anna's bed and holds her hand, then leans back and watches TV with her for a few minutes. While Anna snuggles up to him, Evonne keeps a respectful distance, but he never leaves her sight. After a while, Evonne says, "Anna has school tomorrow. She may want to get to bed."

"Good night, Daddy. I love you. Good night, Evonne," Anna says cheerfully. Hugh leaves the room with his personal guardian.

On Thursday, Hugh and I meet with his occupational therapist, Penny, at HealthSouth. She wants to review shower safety with both of us. I tell her about Hugh feeling faint. "He should not get up quickly from bed—sit first, then stand," she advises. "I think these spells are caused by his systolic blood pressure."

"It happens when he shaves too," I say.

She looks at Hugh and continues. "Try sitting down while you shave, see if that helps. When you're standing, the back and forth motion while looking in the mirror can throw off your equilibrium." Hugh nods agreeably at her.

We also decide to invest in a shower seat and hand-held shower device. I mention that Hugh never wants to shower. Penny turns to Hugh and cocks her head. "Why don't you want to take a shower?" she asks.

"It's too cold," he says.

"Well, suck it up and take one anyway." Hugh's eyebrows shoot up. He breaks into a wide grin. "Suck it up" was a phrase he used all the time in bike racing.

I am advised to accompany Hugh at all times and stay close by while he is in the bathroom. He hates this and so do I, but slipping poses a risk to his compression site, especially in the shower. In protest, he locks me out of the bathroom one morning, propelling me into a panic.

"Are you okay in there?" I call through the door. "Please don't lock me out. What if you feel lightheaded again?"

"I'm fine, leave me alone," he shouts back.

"I can't leave you alone, Hugh, I'm supposed to stay with you in case you feel dizzy."

"I'm fine. Leave me alone. I don't need you."

"Remember the dent in your head, Hugh? You need to be careful not to fall."

"I won't fall, I'm fine." My shoulder is pressed up against the door and I'm beginning to get really peeved. Finally, he unlocks the door and we talk things out calmly. He agrees not to lock the door if I promise to wait outside. A few hours later, we test this out. Within minutes I ask, "Are you okay?"

"Don't rush me," he warns.

Once done with safety issues, Penny works on Hugh's writing. His first exercise is to write down the names of the states where he has lived, using his left hand. She walks away and says she'll be right back to check his work. He begins to write slowly: "VT, NY." He's abbreviating. Glancing up, he sees that Penny is out of sight and switches to his right hand, penning furiously, "FL, VA." *His reasoning is damaged? My foot!*

"You cheater," I whisper to him.

He looks up and says, "So?" I can see he's wondering if I'll tell on him. His eyes search my face to see if I'll be a willing co-conspirator. I have to hold back my smile. Penny figures out his tricks right away without any help from me. She gives him more work and he playfully complains. Like a cat, he morphs from sly to charming in an instant, anything to get his way.

I had written to my parents that Hugh was beginning to read again. While it's slow and he isn't retaining all of it, he's improving steadily. He used to read a book in one or two nights. My parents must have put the word out, because the doorbell rings and it's UPS with a box from my brother, Bill, and his wife, Cindy. It contains a subscription to the *Wall St. Journal* and several food gifts marked, "From one chocoholic to another." Hugh digs right into the cookies and chocolate.

On Friday morning, we're running late as usual. The taxi arrives early, I'm behind on a résumé job, need to pick up the shower stool, and the insurance company needs a fax, but our fax machine is broken. Oddly, I'm in a good mood anyway thinking about the bizarre start of my day. When I went into the bathroom Hugh called out, "You okay in there? I better come watch you shower! You might slip!" The music of his laughter still rings in my ears.

Chapter 20

God placed you in my path.

-Leane, the nurse at the accident scene

I think more and more about the accident that began all this. Suddenly I feel an overwhelming urge to know what happened in the first few moments that brought us to this place. I still have the phone number of Leane, the nurse who was at the scene on the day of the accident. At four o'clock, I nervously dial. She answers immediately, sounding tired. "Hello. This is Rosemary Rawlins," I say. "Are you the woman who helped a cyclist at a car accident on Nuckols Road in early April?"

"Yes! Yes, that's me. I'm so glad you called. How are you? How is your husband?"

"He's getting better, but it's been tough. I'm sorry it took so long for me to call. I just didn't know if I could handle knowing what it was like that day."

"It was chaos. I wanted so much to help him, but he couldn't really talk to me. I saw he was married…the ring. I wondered about you, worried about you," she says. "I heard you have twin girls."

"We do. We'd all love to meet you in person, especially Hugh."

"I can come tomorrow, if you want. I can't wait to lay eyes on him again, and to meet you and your girls," she says. I hang up the phone as Hugh returns from rehab looking completely spent. He's drenched, wearing sweats, and it's near ninety outside.

"A cool shower might feel good," I say.

"No, no shower," he moans. I barely get a half of a sandwich and some Motrin into him when he falls into a deep sleep. His scalp is a mass of dandruff and the skin on his neck is peeling off in sheets. I am dying to soak him in dandruff shampoo. I'm also jealous of his ability to sleep anywhere when I can find no rest and my head is splitting.

"We'll try the new handheld shower later," I whisper to my sleepy husband. A while later, he wakes up and with coaxing, agrees to shower.

Hugh sits on the shower stool. As I'm handing him the shower massage, he grabs it from me and pulls the shower curtain shut so tight I can't see in. I wait on the other side of the blue fabric drape and hear the gentle water cascading around him. All of a sudden, there's a new noise—the rat-tat-tat of water shooting out like machinegun fire. He has changed the setting on the shower massage to "jet/pulse" and it's blasting out in hard streams.

"Hugh, don't put that near your head!" I yank the shower curtain open, causing a blast of cold air, so he grabs it from me again and pulls it shut.

"Hugh, that shooting water will hurt your head!" I tear open the curtain and pull the shower massage from him to readjust it. Heart hammering, I imagine the jet stream of water blowing a hole right through his compression site.

"Oh, I didn't think of that," he says looking up at me with sopping wet hair and stuck together eyelashes.

"Keep it on *spray*, please!" I say. But now the sight of him sitting naked on a stool looking so small and vulnerable suddenly makes me want to hold him in my arms and cry for both of us.

"Okay. I'm fine. Leave me alone." The curtain shuts again. I turn around to the sink and see my pale face in the mirror. I breathe deeply to slow the adrenaline rush and lean against the counter to get my bearings before helping him finish.

"I'm going to wash your head, now," I say, leaning inside the shower. He jumps when I squirt shampoo on his head. After rinsing off, I tell him it's time to come out.

"Shut the curtain! It's cold out there," he says. Again I wait. "Want me to warm up the towel in the dryer?" I offer to get him out. I run down the hall and when I come back, he steps into the warm towel and casually says, "That was nice but the shampoo was a little cold. Next time could you nuke the shampoo?"

"Sorry. No. That's where I draw the line!" Ah, the brain-injured spa life, I think.

Even after being washed, Hugh's head is in nasty shape. Constant itching has caused him to ask for his "do rag" on more than one occasion. To him, this is any piece of fabric, the rougher, the better. He'll rub a dishtowel or washcloth on his head to relieve the itch without scratching. Once he is done rubbing, he simply lets the rag sit on his head all askew. The girls and I walk by and roll our eyes at this new quirk. We have stopped asking questions.

On Saturday morning, Leane pulls up in front of the house right on time. Before she reaches the mailbox, the girls and I run to meet her. Instinctively we exchange hugs. She is young and beautiful with a wild mass of wavy auburn hair. Hugh is waiting in his recliner. Leane approaches him and he shakily stands for a hug. She steps back and takes a good look at him before sitting down. I am not sure she can reconcile the man she saw in the road with him now. His tan is gone, his head is dented, and he's lost a good portion of his body weight.

She tells her story of that day while staring at Hugh the whole time as if in disbelief. Hugh is touched but confused. He has no recollection of the accident. "I don't remember," he says. "It's like hearing about someone else."

"It is an absolute miracle that you are alive," she says to him.

"I must have thought I died and went to heaven when I saw you," he says. Leane laughs, and I say, "Okay, Casanova, that's enough!"

Hugh's parents arrive at the house and thank Leane with firm hugs. Before she leaves, I ask her to write in my journal. She sits quietly in the dining room and records her thoughts:

May 25, 2002
Hugh,

After an extended visit to the hardware store with my husband, God placed you in my path. You had an accident and there were others who stopped as well. We were concerned for you and your family. You and I kept talking about all kinds of things so you wouldn't drift asleep. I remember your sky blue eyes looking at me as if to say don't let me go, keep trying and find my wife. I saw your wedding ring and at that moment, I was on a mission to locate your family. God had his plan in motion and all things were in place. The man who found your cell phone pushed the right buttons and the rescue squad made the right decisions and you fought long and hard to be back at home and I'm so proud of you and are amazed at your progress. I hope we all remain connected. You have changed many lives."

In the afternoon, Jim comes by to mow the lawn and have lunch with Hugh. Electra later visits and surprises Hugh with a long massage when he says his back feels tight. She works on him for an hour and shows me reflexology, demonstrating how rubbing the big toe in circles helps relieve headaches. Wrapping up, she tells Hugh she will return every week to give him a free massage. He flashes me a big smile when she turns to go.

Before bed, Hugh picks up my journal and flips to Leane's page. "It's weird that she says I changed many lives. What do you think she meant by that?"

"I know you changed my life more than once since I married you!" I say.

I can see by his face that he's not so sure how to take that, but he pulls me close anyway.

Chapter 21

May 26, 2002

Dear Hugh,

Right now, I am remembering your wedding day in the backyard tent – and how happy I was to be a part of it. You two were a perfect couple then and through the years your love has grown deeper and you have both managed to look no older in the process. Maybe there is something in the water down there in Virginia! At the risk of embarrassing your wife, when she visited me last summer with the girls, I couldn't help noticing how she still beamed that beautiful smile of hers whenever she mentioned your name. I remember specifically how she confessed that you still managed to push her buttons after all these years. I know that this love you two share will get you through the tough days ahead as you get back on your feet. Meanwhile, just know that you have quite a support team working around you who are all anxious to see that handsome smile of yours soon.

Donna

> \- Rosemary's high school friend

Six weeks out

Once again, Evonne takes off Saturday night to see if Hugh's night prowling has become manageable for us. It is his second week home. Mary and I decide to take turns staying with him while the other one sleeps. Staying awake to watch Hugh is not an option for Anna who easily nods off and could sleep through a tornado. Mary and I each manage two to three hours of sleep on Saturday night, which feels more like an interrupted nap than a good night's rest. We catch each other yawning all morning.

Keith is coming today to preside over the renewal of our wedding vows so I can replace the repaired ring back on Hugh's finger. I had arranged for this on impulse earlier in the week with a quick phone call. Keith was eager to oblige—no company, no party—just a simple promise before God with our children as witnesses.

Our morning is taken up with rearranging the bedroom. We set up a green wooden drop leaf table as a grooming station for Hugh with Mary's old purple mirror hanging above it and a Queen Anne dining room chair tucked underneath. We use the plastic basin provided by the hospital for a portable sink. Hugh can now sit to shave and brush his teeth without dizziness. The whole set-up proves tacky but functional.

We also move Mary's twin bed next to our queen bed to create a makeshift king-sized bed. On Evonne's nights off, I have found Hugh to be a restless sleeper, and this arrangement will give us more room. While Mary and I transfer beds, Anna plays cards with Hugh. This is a far cry from the morning of pampering I enjoyed at the beauty parlor before my first wedding.

Keith Emerson arrives early in the afternoon following Sunday service at Epiphany to preside over our ceremony. Dark half moon dents underline my eyes and Hugh has chocolate crumbs on his lips from a cookie he has just eaten, but it doesn't matter, I dust him off. Keith chats as I pull a kitchen chair beside Hugh's recliner. Dressed in a denim skirt and summer top, I repeat the vows I made almost twenty-five years ago. Mary and Anna stand nearby and watch as our new marriage unites our past to a present more incredible than we had ever imagined. Our eyes connect as we hear the words, "Will you love him, comfort him, honor and keep him, in sickness and in health; and, forsaking all others, be faithful to him as long as you both shall live?" I see a glimpse of Hugh's old soul as I place his ring back on his weak left hand. When I let go, his fingers fall on the chair's arm like a series of oblong weights. I wonder: will he ever take care of me again—in sickness—in health?

Once our rings are secured, we join hands with Keith, Mary, and Anna, and recite the Lord's Prayer. As we open our eyes, Keith lifts the small box of wafers he has brought along and serves each of us communion. When the ceremony is finished, he steps back with a smile, and says, "This has been one of the high points of my priesthood."

"I never really planned on getting married again," Hugh says, and we all laugh.

To me, this ceremony is my acceptance of the radically changed circumstances of our marriage. I am dedicating myself not only to Hugh, but to whatever lies ahead for us together. I see from their faces that Anna and Mary sense the immensity of this moment. Our children have witnessed us saying our wedding vows while watching us live them.

By late afternoon, my eyes burn with exhaustion. Mary is planning to spend the night at a friend's house and I am counting the hours until Evonne comes. I fantasize about thick cotton bed sheets and a soft pillow. When the phone rings, I walk so slowly that I barely make it before the answering machine picks up. It's Evonne. "Mrs. Rawlins I am so sorry," she says, "but I had to mow thirty acres today with a push mower and I am just too tired to stay awake all night with Mr. Rawlins this evening. You know I don't want to fall asleep accidentally, so I better not come."

"Oh." I'm shocked into silence. "It's okay, Evonne," I finally choke out. "We'll be fine."

"Again, I'm so sorry. I don't want to be too tired to keep a good eye on him."

"I understand," I say, and slowly hang up the phone, lean over the desk, and burst into tears. I cannot stay awake the entire night again. My stomach rolls with nausea. The phone rings almost immediately again and Mary answers from upstairs. She shouts down to me, "Mom, it's for you." *What now?* I wonder.

"Hi Rosemary, it's Electra. How's Hugh's back today?"

"He's better today."

"What's wrong? You sound terrible."

"Mary and I have been up most of the night and Evonne just called to say she can't come to sit with Hugh tonight. I don't want Mary to have to cancel her sleepover plans to back me up. It seems she can never just be a kid."

Electra knows I'm at my wit's end. "Let me come. You can go to bed. It'll be fun—I'll bring a few videos to watch."

I don't argue with her. "Let me come," she says, as if I were doing *her* a favor. She shows up promptly at eight and sits upstairs in the back room with Hugh. I hear them laughing as I walk back to my bedroom. I fall asleep upon impact with the pillow and don't wake up until two a.m. Disoriented at first, I turn over, then remember Electra and shuffle back to the guest room where she is sitting patiently in Evonne's high back chair. An immense wave of love fills me as she signals me over. She tells me Hugh has slept on and off—once he was restless, so she gave him a massage to help him sleep. Here it is, the night of my second wedding, and I have let my husband spend the night with another woman, a beautiful masseuse no less! The thought makes me giggle.

"Thank you, Electra. I feel much better. I'm sure I can get through the rest of the night with him." After hugging her at the front door, I slip into bed beside Hugh and listen to the sound of his rhythmic breathing.

Memorial Day is no day off for Hugh—he has rehab. He usually refuses to shave, but this morning, he removes his goatee to please Anna. "You look so handsome, Dad," she tells him. The cab picks him up early, as usual. The girls both have plans with friends. I have an entire morning to myself, so I decide to go to the swim club.

Lying in the sun in my bathing suit, I try to read, but I keep thinking of all the summer days we spent at the pool as a family when the girls were little. The girls and I would arrive at the pool early afternoon and Hugh would arrive after work in his business suit, grab a pair of shorts from the car trunk, and change in the locker room. Anna and Mary would dive off Hugh's shoulders or he would swim under water and pull their toes as they kicked. We were all involved in swim team. I can hear him yelling, "Go Mary Lou, Go Goose," as the race began and they dove off the blocks. We ate grilled hamburgers and junk food from the cake sale and stayed late into the night.

I sit at the pool and wonder if he will ever walk on the coping without slipping again or get in and out of the lap pool without help. I wonder if he will be able to swim with his weak left arm. He was once an ocean lifeguard and a competitive sailor and surfer.

"Hi Rosemary. Mind if I sit here?" It's Celeste, a friend of mine. She lays her towel on a chaise and sets her canvas bag on the patio. She looks sideways at me from under a big floppy hat.

"No, not at all," I say. "How are the kids? Will they do swim team?" I haven't talked to Celeste in weeks. I'm out of touch with most of my friends. I know she's kept up with Hugh's progress through her husband, Rich, who had come by the hospital often to check on us since he works nearby. She fills me in on her family, while sensitively treading away from hospital talk. Instinctively she knows I'm here to escape, if just for an hour. It feels good to sit by the pool and talk to a friend. It feels so normal.

A sign that hung on the door outside the ICU said, "Normal is a setting on the washing machine." What is normal, really? Was Hugh normal yesterday and suddenly not normal today? Who on earth determines that? Much of what we call normal is just a façade anyway—the way people all dress and act alike, doing and wearing whatever is in style. We are all just who we are, nothing more...or less.

While I rest at the pool, Larry Piper meets Hugh for lunch at HealthSouth. Later he relays his comical mid-day excursion to me. Larry didn't see Hugh in the cafeteria, so he went outside in the courtyard to find him. All the shady tables were occupied and Hugh sat at the only one in direct sun because it was the warmest. There he was with his helmet on, in his sweat pants and sweatshirt, literally baking, but perfectly content. Larry sat across from him and said he nearly passed out from heat exhaustion during lunch.

"Oh, I forgot to mention that the little thermostat in Hugh's brain is temporarily out of order," I tell him, laughing.

Tonight is our first post-injury Memorial Day cookout with Hugh's parents. Ever since Hugh has come home from the hospital he has been fairly sedentary, but tonight he is wired. First he wants to go out on the deck, so we all file out after him. I have his gait belt in my hand. He sits for only a minute and wants to go back inside. "Let go of me," he grumbles, "I can walk," and since it's only about three steps to his chair, I let go. He doesn't go to the chair. Instead, he stands and thinks a minute, then clomps around the kitchen. I lean in to grab his belt again and he snaps at me, "I said I could walk. I want to go outside."

No use telling him he was outside thirty seconds ago. Our picnic is shaping up to be a test of nerves. No one can relax. His parents don't know how to react. Should they help him or let him be? Hugh's father turns burgers and franks on the grill. Hugh tries to take the large fork from him. "You relax, Hugh. Sit on the bench," his father says. Hugh looks peeved but does not talk back. He doesn't sit down either. His eyes dart around suspiciously.

"Where are the girls?" Hugh asks. I point at the glass door. Back inside, the girls are watching television as they scarf down a bag of potato chips with their sodas. Hugh stumbles around the room with me close behind. Everyone tries to act casual, but tension has a way of steaming out into the atmosphere where we all feel it, making Hugh more and more agitated. Finally, we are seated at the table to eat. Hugh rises again. He seems to want to do things to help—to be a host in his house, but he doesn't know what to do. We go through the motions of eating at a quiet dinner table. The hamburger is hard for Hugh to manage and he's covered in bits of food.

After dinner, I shepherd everyone into the living room for a coffee table dessert, hoping to get Hugh into his recliner, but he trips. His mother lets out a loud scream. He stumbles and nearly hits his head on the fireplace but catches himself and falls into his safe chair. His mother gasps, "By Jiminies!" With rattled nerves, we eat our ice cream. Shortly after, Hugh's father grabs his hat. "I think we should be going now," he says. As Hugh struggles to get up out of the chair, his father holds his shoulder down. "You don't have to get up. Get some rest. I love you," he says. He places his plaid bucket hat over his forehead, hiding his eyes, and leaves with Rita, shoulders slumped.

Hugh is trying hard to be normal. It is a question he asks his therapists again and again: "When will I be normal?"

I think about the pre-injury Hugh. That Hugh was smart, athletic, confident, serious, introverted, devoted to his family, loyal to his friends. He was generous to those he loved, but not easy to get to know, and quiet in a crowd. Those who did not know him well sometimes mistook his quiet demeanor and serious look for indifference or aggravation. He was not interested in impressing anyone and never faked his emotions. But if he loved you, you knew it. It was wonderful to be loved by Hugh, like gaining membership to an exclusive club. Since the accident, this open side of him has become more prominent. He is now more extraverted and impulsive, he laughs easily, and smiles more. Some of our friends have commented that he's easier to talk to now and they welcome the change. Interestingly, it's his sharper edge the girls and I miss.

"I miss being scared of Daddy," Mary says to me one night.

"I do too. He's different now, but I have a feeling he'll be more like himself again someday. It will just take time." I hug her close and hope I am not making false promises.

Nancy Hendrickson, our old neighbor and an R.N., drives us to Hugh's first primary care doctor's visit. Nancy doesn't act different around Hugh as many others do. Some people raise their voice during conversation as if he's hearing impaired. Others look sad in his presence. Nancy jokes with Hugh in the car. After seeing our family doctor, we drop Hugh at rehab and Nancy takes me out to Starbucks. Settling into a couple of deep cozy armchairs in a sunny corner, we savor our lattes and talk. She explains that she has first-hand experience with brain injury. Her mother-in-law had suffered a similar injury in a car accident years ago. She said she was never the same but has learned to adapt and lives a very happy life.

The words: "never the same" keep following me. It is a phrase I hear over and over again about TBI. I have searched the stacks in libraries for stories about brain injury. I flip to the end to see the outcome, only to learn that "things are never the same again" in every story I've read. A few books written by TBI survivors made me weep at the end, because they wrote that life is now radically changed but they have found peace. This seems like a nice way of saying, "life as you know it is over." It is a reality I am only beginning to accept. TBI is a life-changing condition, and yet in almost all the cases, years later, these changes turn out to be viewed as positive ones. I cannot help but wonder what is in store for us. What happens in the interim years as you wait for the positive metamorphosis to occur? We are on day forty-four of this journey, yet it feels like a lifetime already, and I've aged a decade in less than two months.

Hugh still has trouble getting up in the mornings and the girls and

I have had a few highly emotional encounters with him over it. Finally, one morning I have had it after the fourth round of, "Give me fifteen more minutes." Mary and Anna are in tears watching us go through this aggravating scene. They try to intervene but it doesn't work, and they have to leave for school. Once they are gone, in a fit of exasperation, I lose my temper and yell at him.

"You are being so childish. If you don't get up, I won't answer the door. You can explain to everyone at HealthSouth why you aren't ready. I'm sick of this and I'm over it! It's all on you now!" I slam the door and storm downstairs, full of remorse for how I have just acted. I begin crying uncontrollably but pull myself together when I hear him up and moving. He snubs me on his way out the door, his feelings hurt. As the taxi pulls away, I call his occupational therapist, Penny.

"I feel awful. Hugh would not get up this morning and I screamed at him."

"Is this the first time you yelled at him?" she asks me almost disbelieving.

"Yes, I think so," I reply.

"Congratulations. That's pretty good. But it's not right. He really can't help it. Maybe you should talk to someone about dealing with all this."

She suggests I contact HealthSouth's Licensed Clinical Social Worker, Nancy Foley, to talk things out. I agree to call her. I am in way over my head. "For better or for worse, for richer or poorer, in sickness and in health…" I had pledged in my renewal of wedding vows only days ago. This is my new beginning. I need to find my way out of the past and move on.

Do you take this man?

I do.

Chapter 22

Seven weeks out

The cherished sleep provided by Ambien is still my body's only time to recharge. I look forward to Evonne coming like a child anticipating Santa's arrival. I hope I'm not becoming emotionally dependent on sleeping pills. I keep this in check by not taking any pills on the weekends when Evonne takes one or two nights off. I don't sleep on those nights at all, no matter how worn out I am. It's as though my mind is a separate entity from my body, constantly poking and prodding it awake. While I can function all day, something strange happens to me at night when I close my eyes in bed. My heart thumps in my chest and I feel the force of rushing blood drumming in my ears making me want to leap up instead of sleep.

My older brother, John, a scientist, once mused that perhaps each person is born with a genetically predisposed number of heartbeats to expend in their lifetime. It would then be advantageous to have a slow heart rate, and he used that theory to justify not wanting to exercise—he was prolonging his own life by keeping his pulse low. But now I feel a pang of fear that I am burning through my life at breakneck speed, as quickly as a sparkler that flares and fizzles out.

In Hugh's May 30th team meeting, the physical therapist's goal is to see Hugh walk the treadmill for ten minutes without left foot drop. His weak left leg makes his foot drag along the floor and trips him up when he's tired. When he concentrates, he can control it. His other goals in PT include improving balance, walking five hundred feet on a level surface, and up and down steps at a modified independent level. Hugh's occupational therapist states three goals: attend to task, print legibly, and shower independently. Hugh is reported to be exhibiting mild frustration at left hand dexterity and control. His scores on the amnesia test were 65-74, still below the normal range for post-traumatic amnesia. Positives are reported too. His attention span holds for ten minutes without difficulty during a thirty-minute session, not much gain, but improving. He is said to be cooperative and showing progress in a few areas such as orientation; he is consistently aware of the correct month and year. But there is still a long way to go.

It's a warm spring evening and the girls have plans to go out, so Hugh and I invite Kevin to come have dinner with us. Over a meal of rotisserie chicken and vegetables, Kevin asks Hugh what he's been doing lately. Hugh talks about some of his activities at rehab but admits he does little around the house. He will occasionally walk outside around the yard, but not far, and always with me by his side holding his gait belt. After dinner, Kevin suggests he and Hugh go for a walk. At about five feet, nine inches, Kevin is not particularly tall; however, he is broadly and solidly built. Every inch of him is muscle. He has thick thighs and arms and an authoritative voice. He notices me helping Hugh with his socks and sneakers, raises his eyebrows and says, "Let him do that."

I glance up at him. "He says he can't."

Kevin is not convinced. He turns to Hugh. "What do you mean you can't? C'mon, try it." Hugh explains that he cannot bend over, his hamstrings are too tight and he feels dizzy when he puts his head down. Kevin suggests a strategy. While Hugh is sitting in a kitchen chair, he instructs Hugh to lift and rest his right foot on another chair. It is slow, but it takes the pressure off Hugh's hamstring and he is now looking across rather than down so he doesn't feel lightheaded. He puts on his own socks and sneakers by himself for the first time. A slight smile curls up on the right side of his face. I still have to tie them for him because his left hand cannot grasp a shoelace. I ask Hugh, "What does it feel like to be you right now?"

"I feel like I'm in a third dimension. Sometimes I don't know if I'm dreaming or awake," he says, standing and turning toward the front door, his helmet firmly secured to his head. Kevin holds the gait belt to steady him. The two men walk down the steps and out of the cul-de-sac side by side. I hear Kevin's jovial voice fade down the block.

While Kevin and Hugh disappear around the corner, I clean the dinner dishes. The guys are gone for over thirty minutes when I begin to think Hugh fell or was too exhausted to make it home. Though I know that Kevin is perfectly capable, I keep looking out the window. Finally I give up and sit on the front steps until I hear them laughing in the distance. As they round the corner of the cul-de-sac, I see that Hugh is clearly having a great time. They approach the steps smiling and I hold back tears. Together, we amble around the house and stop in the backyard so Hugh can rest in a lawn chair. Kevin asks about the patch of black-eyed-susans and our herb garden, and tells us about the new garden he's putting in.

Once inside, Kevin tells me I'm doing too much for Hugh. "He needs to work harder than ever to get his left side back, and it will require constant work," he says. "It's time you pull away a little, Rosemary. Hugh's a tough guy. He can manage." Noticing my sad face, he adds, "Hang in there," and squeezes my arm.

By the front door, he talks to Hugh. "Hugh, remember how you used to torture me before a race? You were relentless, but you always brought out the best in me."

Hugh laughs. "You weren't a wuss like some others. You could take it," he says.

"I guess. We've spent a lot of time together in the bike saddle; I figure we've ridden about 80,000 miles together—a lot of miles for a friendship. Stay strong buddy. If anyone can work his way out of this, you can!"

Closing the front door after him, Hugh says to me, "I feel like I can do anything when I'm with Kevin."

Kevin's visit is a turning point for several reasons. We discover that simply taking a long evening walk is enough to help Hugh fall asleep at night and stay asleep. This starts a new routine; we walk every night, no matter what the weather. June 1st is Evonne's last night with Hugh. In the morning, she reports that he slept soundly all the way through. I take photos of him with her as we say our goodbyes. "I'll miss sharing Teddy Grahams with you," she jokes.

When I call Kevin to tell him the good news, he says, "Way to go, Rosemary," like the trainer he is. More softly he says, "Hugh is a mentor to me. I'm glad I could help out."

Recognizing the people that are helping us keeps our family from engaging in a pity party, an easy trap to fall into. A few weeks back, I had taken up a collection for the Fire Station to honor the men who rescued Hugh in April. Friends, relatives, and Hugh's coworkers gave generously. On Sunday morning, I drive the family down Mountain Road to Fire Station 15 to meet Ed Wood, the Lieutenant who was at the accident scene, and some of the men who were on duty that day. When Hugh walks into the station in his baseball cap, shakes each person's hand, and says thank-you, they are blown away. "We truly did not expect you to live through the night," says one fireman, as he shakes Hugh's hand. "I can tell you one thing, you're a fighter. It took nine of us to strap you on that body board. We knew it would take a fighting spirit to get you through this. You surprised even us!"

Hugh's face is a mixture of gratitude, humility, and curiosity. He whispers to me that hearing about his rescue is like hearing about another person, but this is the closest he's felt to experiencing it. After Ed Wood shakes Hugh's hand, Hugh tells me it wrapped completely around his, as if his hand was a tiny child's. "That man is strong!" he says. Ed is several inches taller than Hugh, a human bear, only he's gregarious instead of dangerous. "I can't believe you didn't get me into the ambulance all by yourself," Hugh says to Ed, with a look of mock fear. "Why would I want to fight *you*?" The men laugh.

"We're just glad you made it through," says Ed. Looking at Anna and Mary he adds, "Looks like you had a few good reasons!" The girls present the men with our gift basket and I give each man a copy of our letter of thanks before we snap pictures of them with Hugh by the fire truck.

"Now that was amazing!" Hugh says all the way home. While he looks genuinely pleased, I feel a mix of emotion, a sappy sense of happiness and sadness all at once.

Our life is a sitcom, tragedy, and drama rolled into one. My emotions come in waves—sometimes they crash, sometimes they shine as smooth as glass. My mood can change in a minute. I waffle between denial and acceptance, anger and peace, or joy and sorrow at the slightest provocation. I have learned that it is possible to feel two conflicting emotions at the same time. I feel lucky and cheated, thankful and ungrateful, hopeful and hopeless.

The small things make me cry: an act of kindness when I don't expect it, a gesture Hugh makes that is familiar from our past. But sometimes I weep at any bleak reminder that our lives have radically changed. One morning, while out on errands, I feel particularly happy. The sun is shining in a cloudless cobalt sky. Hugh has gotten up early and is with a friend before rehab, so I have a few morning hours alone. I'm light-hearted, riding in the car singing an oldie with the Lovin' Spoonful on the radio. My trip to the post office is perfect, no line today. Driving back toward the grocery store, I pass my own neighborhood and notice a taxi pull out behind me—Hugh's taxi—driving him to rehab. The cab pulls up alongside me at the red light, and there in the back seat sits my 46-year-old husband buckled up like a child, waving to me with a crooked smile and a big clumsy helmet strapped on his head. I drive to the far end of the nearest empty parking lot and sob.

"It's time to pull back, Rosemary," Kevin had said. How? How can I do that now?

I meet Nancy Foley for the first time with reserve. She is the social worker Penny suggested, the one who helps patients and families cope while they are at HealthSouth. I have never been to a counselor before. I'm afraid of opening the valve to my thoughts, afraid to see what gushes out. What if I'm as crazy as I feel?

All of my reservations are swept away as Nancy greets me with warmth in her homey office with its beautiful pictures, inspirational sayings, and comfortable furniture. "Thanks for seeing me," I begin. She welcomes me in, gestures toward a fabric-covered chair, and gets right to the point.

"How are you, Rosemary?"

"I'm fine." Nancy's eyebrows go up. I shift in my chair, and look at her. She's petite, conservatively dressed in button down blouse, slacks, and sensible flat shoes, but my sixth sense tells me she's tuned in, that she can see right through me. "Hugh seems to be a little better," I say flatly. Nancy tilts her head as if she didn't hear me correctly. "Things are going well." Now she knows I'm either lying or in serious denial. I quickly change the subject to divert attention from myself. "What a beautiful picture that is…"

Just as agile, Nancy zooms in on me. "But, how are *you* doing, Rosemary? You haven't told me about *you*."

"Oh, I'm fine." My shoulders stiffen.

"Really?"

"Well, no…" My eyes fill up.

"What's on your mind?"

I can't speak. *Everything. Everything's on my mind! I can't even find my mind there's so much stuff on it! And we only have twenty-eight minutes left to talk. How do I put it all into words?* She reads my face.

"You must feel overwhelmed."

Overwhelmed doesn't even scratch the surface. "My life's a mess! I don't know where to begin…this could take years," I try to joke. My words drift pathetically through the air. Nancy nods reassuringly.

"Everything's different now—my husband, my house, my job. I hardly ever see the kids. Friends are driving them. I can't sleep. I don't want to socialize. I just feel so alone!"

"Rosemary, what you are feeling is completely understandable," she says. "But let's break things down. What bothered you today?"

"Hugh just won't get up and get going. It's a battle every day. I'm tired of arguing with him."

"Okay. Describe to me what your morning was like today."

"Well, don't forget, Hugh has TBI, two teenage girls, and I'm premenopausal, so I'm sure it's no picnic for him either."

"What happened today?"

"I tell Hugh it's time to get up. He asks for a few more minutes. A short while later, I say it's time for rehab. He says he's getting up, but he's not. He's hunkering down in the pillow." Nancy smiles. I know she can picture his face. "I hear Mary scream from the bathroom in frustration, and Anna's yelling, 'Hurry up, we'll be late!' I walk across the hall and find Mary with a ponytail elastic tangled in her hair, and do the only thing I can do to fix it fast. I grab my scissors and cut the knot out. She screams that I cut too much hair. Meanwhile, Anna's still yelling, 'Hurry up, Mary, the bus!' Mary jumps down the stairs, two at a time, and they leave for the bus stop. I walk back into the bedroom where Hugh's still in bed. I try to hold on to my temper, 'Hugh, it's time to get up.' I know I sound mad, but I can't help it. I know he's tired. I know he's sick. I just can't help being frustrated..."

"Go on, it's okay to feel angry," she says.

"So, Hugh says, 'I *am* getting up. Can you stop bugging me?' like I'm some kind of annoying fly, and not his wife. 'You are NOT getting up—you're still in bed!' I say, pretty loud. I hear the front door slam down stairs. It's the girls again, all out of breath. They scream up to me, 'Mom, we missed the bus. Can you drive us?' By now, I'm frazzled. Hugh's still in bed so I say to him, 'Okay now, Hugh, time to get *out* of bed!' He gives me this *grin* and pushes the covers back. He knows by my face, it's not a good time to push his luck. He shuffles to the bathroom—so slow, it kills me. We hear Anna yell that the taxi is here."

Nancy rolls her eyes and shakes her head with an air of horrified amusement. Something about her makes me want to gush out my angst like a torrent from a hydrant.

"We all dive in rushing Hugh through his routine. I yell to the girls, 'Mary, stall the cab. Anna, find Dad's sneakers. I grab his notebook and reading glasses, smooth his hair, and guide him out the door toward the taxi driver. Then I remember I need to write a résumé by noon. I have papers to fax, and the girls are yelling at me to hurry, they'll be late for school, so I ignore the cramps in my stomach, grab my keys, and hold my tongue. We pack into the Explorer and drive to school, turning into the parking lot just in time for first block. *This* is what I mean by starting the day off wrong. We seem to be out of control most days," I say, breathing hard. Nancy listens. I can't stop. I look at the floor and keep speaking.

"I drive back home to the empty house and scream out loud in the foyer like some crazy woman in a movie, just to let out the pressure building inside me! I call my client and postpone my résumé meeting. I can't concentrate, no work today. Then I drive here, hoping to God I won't crash from all the distraction in my brain."

Nancy sits straight in her chair. "That's quite a morning," she says. "And I can see you're frustrated. We can work with Hugh here by talking about getting ready for rehab. At home, try setting alarms, more than one maybe. Shift the burden of waking up to him. Or, have a friend call him to wake him up. We'll get more ideas from Penny."

Nancy's suggestion makes me think of Kevin. If Kevin called Hugh in the morning, I bet he'd get up, or Lee, maybe Lee. I tell Nancy it's overwhelming to have everyone ask what's going on all the time—even though they are asking out of love and concern. I hate to not answer them, but I feel like I have been swallowed by Hugh's injury, I'm in the belly of it, churning around. I can't fight my way out.

Nancy advises me to pick two or three trusted friends. "Tell them everything. Confide in them. Get it out of your system, but then let it go. The rest of the world does not need to know everything. You can't live this every minute of every day by retelling the details of your life to each and every person."

Nancy gives me direction without telling me I am overprotective or overreacting. To my surprise, she says I am intellectualizing too much and not emoting enough! I know then and there that I have a very active, loud and emphatic internal life! I have running dialogs in my head all the time—and boy, they are emoting loud and clear! She wants me to let them out, but it's like a clogged pipe.

"You never asked for this to happen, Rosemary, but it has, and you have a right to be angry and feel cheated. You never even had time to grieve and recover from the trauma of Hugh's accident and those days in the hospital because you've been too busy. It's not easy and it's going to be trial and error for a while. Be gentle with yourself and gentle with Hugh. You are two strong people with a lot of love between you— that's very plain to see. Take each minute for what it is and try to move forward without expectations for the long run. Things will work out in time."

Nancy tells me it is common for the spouse of someone with a brain injury to feel a deep sense of grief as if that spouse had *died*. The word, though spoken calmly, jolts me like an unexpected thunderclap. I had been thinking this myself and pushed the thought away; I didn't dare verbalize it. Hugh *didn't* die. And yet I hardly know him anymore. His eyes are vacant. Our communication system is severed. There's no way to grieve, mourn or explain the void I feel inside. People always say to me, "Isn't it a miracle that he survived that crash?"

Did he?

This very thought is compounded by guilt because he's still living; he's just drastically changed in demeanor and appearance, here in body, but not in mind or spirit. On one level, I love him more than ever, more deeply than I thought I ever could, and at the same time, I'm not sure I know him anymore.

Nancy assures me that more of the Hugh I knew will surface, aspect by aspect. Each familiar emergence will be precious, though some of his new personality traits may be confusing or scary. "Building a new rewarding relationship requires flexibility and a willingness to accept change," she says. "It will take work on the part of both of you to create a new kind of relationship, especially now while he's healing, but I have no doubt that you both have the will and desire to do that."

Nancy's tender words are followed by some sobering news: "It's not going to be easy. You'll have to work hard. Many relationships fail after a brain injury due to unrealistic expectations or fear of the future."

I make up my mind that ours will not.

Chapter 23

Dear Anna and Mary
Sorry about your dad's accident. I baked you these cookies to cheer you up a
little. I hope it works. Thinking of you.
Your friend,
Mickey

-Mickey Vetter, Anna and Mary's school friend

Eight weeks out

66"Time to get up," I say. Hugh rises without complaint and trudges toward the bathroom. He hits the doorjamb with his left shoulder and grunts. At least I'm not pulling him out of bed anymore. Therapy is paying off. The morning reminder routine begins: "Brush your teeth. Rinse. Spit. Time to shave. Comb your hair. Take your medicine. Put on your helmet." I am narrating his life, repeating each step several times. And if something isn't said, it doesn't get done…day after day after day. I fasten his gait belt and guide him to the door where the taxi driver takes over for rehab.

While Hugh is gone, I rush through chores, clean the house, shop for groceries, and focus on writing the few résumés I've accepted. I feel particularly sluggish today—sluggish but jumpy. It's like I've developed my own attention deficit disorder lately. I move from chore to chore, forgetting what I started in one room as I enter the next, unable to stick to any one thing until it's done. And right in the middle of doing something, I'll remember that I needed to call this doctor or the insurance company—and I wonder what else I didn't remember—and I interrupt myself, losing all concentration for the work I was doing before. Today I decide I need a master To Do list. I need to see even the smallest accomplishment ticked off in black ink. I need some verification of progress!

While composing my list, I hear widely spaced, thudding footsteps on the porch signaling that Hugh's cab driver is guiding him up to our front door after rehab. "These are for you," he says handing me papers from his speech therapist, Michaelle, as he enters the front door. The papers explain *executive function*, one of the deficits resulting from Hugh's injury to the frontal lobes.

Executive function relates to a person's ability to initiate, plan, fix mistakes, complete, and evaluate the results of any given activity. It affects everything in daily life from cooking to paying the bills. To control behavior, executive function keeps us from blurting out inappropriate thoughts.

Hugh shows significant loss of executive function, but we are told he is making strides every week. I am cautioned about not perceiving Hugh as lazy or unmotivated. These characteristics are a result of his brain injury, and with therapy, time, and compensatory strategies, there may be more improvement. Executive function is part of the reason Hugh spends so much time resting while at home. He often sits in his chair unless I suggest a walk, meal, or some activity. He's not only tired, he's unaware that there are other things he can do.

To understand brain injury, one resident told me to imagine the billions of neurons in my brain as tiny arms holding messages that they pass back and forth to monitor all vital bodily functions (heart rate, breathing, etc.), control the five senses, regulate hormones, and perform every physical, mental, and emotional task. During the injury, some of those arms are amputated (the neurons killed off). Thus, their messages are no longer sent or received. In some cases, the little arm next to an amputated arm decides to change direction and pass its message around the dead one to complete the job – a detour of sorts. This is the brain's ingenious way of healing itself. It's called "building new pathways" and results in some recovery of function.

It doesn't always work, though. Sometimes, the arm is simply gone, and with it, the job it once performed, leaving the person with a deficit, much like a cut phone wire where no message is transmitted. No matter how hard you try or how much you want it, the line is dead. When this is the case, compensatory strategies are put into place to help the person deal with the deficit in practical ways: writing reminder notes, or setting up systems to help them remember where they put things. Some deficits can be helped quite a bit by these strategies; some can't be helped at all.

As I review the papers Hugh brought home, the human resource administrator in me kicks in. I understand the process of hiring and retaining qualified employees. Executive Function is the most serious problem I see regarding Hugh's return to work, especially at the level of Assistant Controller for a large corporation. Accounting requires strict attention to detail. His ability to sustain attention is impaired. He will be seriously challenged when formulating goals, planning work, identifying mistakes, meeting deadlines, and supervising staff. These strengths are all essential in his management position. I am anxious to see him take charge again, to start a project and finish it. He's beginning to do this a little in his morning routine. Although it takes time, he is following the steps necessary to get ready for rehab.

The long list of simple things he can't do will come as a shock to his boss and work associates. I'm sure no one has a realistic sense of how much Hugh is fighting to regain, and I don't want them to know just yet.

Hugh and I sit down to dinner alone. We can hear Mary typing on the computer keyboard in my office just down the hall. In the middle of our quiet meal, Mary screams out, "Mom, come here!" I jump up from the table instinctively and run for the office, not realizing that behind me, Hugh is doing the same. Before I reach the office, Mary and I hear a crash. Both of us rush back to the kitchen where we find Hugh on the floor.

"Dad!" Mary screams. "Are you alright?"

"I guess I just slipped. At least I didn't take it on the head!" he says laughing.

"If you weren't wearing those dorky white socks you wouldn't slip!" Mary jokes.

"It *is* June. You can go barefoot now," I say, smiling at him. As scary as it is that he fell, it's a clear sign he's responding to Mary's call for help, and that's a step forward. "You did a great job breaking your fall. Your arm okay?" I ask helping him up.

"I'm fine, but what was wrong, Mary?" he asks. We both look at her.

"Oh. I found the perfect puppy on the Internet. I wanted to show Mom right away."

"Don't scare me like that again!" Hugh scolds in a playful way. Mary shines with delight that he is regaining his protective nature. Pulling him into my office, she stops him in front of the monitor. "Isn't he the most adorable thing you ever saw?" she sighs. Hugh makes her a promise: "I'll buy you any dog you want when you get your first apartment." Mary is ecstatic, "Really Dad? Really?" Hugh nods his head. This is one off-the-cuff promise he'll really have to keep.

A few times after that, I catch Hugh doing his home assignments from rehab on his own. They involve all kinds of everyday information-gathering, such as looking up telephone numbers in the phone book, finding certain articles in the newspaper, or locating the weather report. In addition, he's given skills worksheets to complete. These range from reading comprehension exercises to simple math problems or other exercises to increase his cognitive speed, such as writing down as many words as he can conjure up that start with a certain letter.

Hugh completes these worksheets and is supposed to take notes while at rehab. He carries a marble composition notebook for that purpose, but never writes a single word in it. He's never been much of a note-taker anyway. The front cover reveals a deep sense of determination, however. On the three blank lines Hugh has written:

Name: Rawlins

School: Hard knocks

Grade: A+

Chapter 24

Rosemary

The girls are dancers and they should dance. Never worry about that. You never have to pay me a penny again or worry about lessons. I know things are difficult right now. I want to keep teaching them – I love your girls. If they need a ride to dance, call and I'll pick them up too.

Love,

Peggy

-Peggy Thibodeau, Owner of Shuffles Dance Studio

Eight weeks out

Poised in pink ballet shoes, with softly curved beckoning arms, Mary says, "When I get married, I want to have ballerinas dance down the aisle ahead of me in the church." Gracefully turning on her toes across the kitchen floor, she breathlessly asks me which series of turns would look prettiest in church. Her hair swirls in shiny waves. She is once again lost in the fantasy of what she calls the most important day of her life. From upstairs, I can hear the rhythmic thumping of Anna's hip-hop music. Now and again a boom resonates on the kitchen ceiling from a jump she has performed in her bedroom. Both girls are eager for their dance recital.

Each year, Peggy produces an impressive production at the historic Landmark Theater in downtown Richmond. Locals call it "the Mosque." The theater was built in 1926 as a spectacular replica of a Moslem temple. Its auditorium seats nearly five thousand people and the rising dome above is adorned with seventy-five thousand square feet of gold leaf. This exotic space provides a lavish set for the end-of-year dance recital, the culminating event for Shuffles dance students and their families.

A lot of planning goes into preparing Hugh to attend this recital. First, we check with the doctors to see if he should go. They point out that the loud noise and length will be issues, but we can compensate for both. I buy him foam earplugs and we plan to have him leave at intermission, figuring he can sit for about two hours.

The girls and I also decide it is time to clean up Hugh's head for his big night out. His last haircut occurred on a gurney in the emergency room when he was prepared for surgery. His hair was hastily chopped off at all different lengths resulting in an irregular Mohawk, a wide stripe of hair down the middle of the back of his head where they didn't bother to shave because it was not part of the operation site. A piece of his skull is still missing, and now the dent in his head has sunken in deep where the swelling on his brain has receded. He also sports many new scars. Anna holds the scissor above his head. "Be very careful," I caution.

"It's easy, Mom, I can do this. I do it all the time on my own hair."

Hugh sits statue-still on a plastic lawn chair on the back deck, a bath towel around his shoulders, squinting in the bright sunshine. Anna snips off a lock of his Mohawk. "Ow!" Hugh yells. Anna jerks away. Hugh laughs and she slaps his shoulder.

"Dad, don't do that. It's not funny! I thought I hurt you." After shaking off the jitters, she tries to even up the longer sides, but finds it hard to navigate between the scabs and scars. We decide to deal with it later. It is passable for now.

Early Saturday morning, Lee calls. He had come by earlier to drive the girls to dress rehearsal so I could stay home with Hugh. "Hey, just thought you should know... the girls are in the *STAR* dressing room. I'm impressed!"

"Pretty cool," I say smiling. Peggy had purposely arranged to have the girls with her, including them for meals between shows to eliminate my having to drive back and forth.

"Yeah, little V.I.P.'s you've got there," he says. I hang up the phone and I'm telling Hugh the news when the doorbell rings. It's Jim.

"I heard you had a fashion emergency," he jokes.

"More like a haircut emergency," I say.

Hugh chimes in, "Ah, just chop it all off." After pulling out the electric trimmer I bought to clean up Hugh's haircut, we settle on a buzz cut. Jim sets the trimmer and shows me how to use it. When we're done, he pulls the drape off Hugh and announces, "There! He's still just as ugly, but at least his hair looks better." Hugh flashes him a lopsided smirk and elbows him in the arm before heading back to the Laz-Z-Boy for a rest.

Jim starts mowing the lawn as Krista arrives from William and Mary College. "Uncle Hugh, you look so much better now. The last time I saw you, you were in the ICU!" Despite the heat, Hugh is dressed in warm clothes as Jim comes in the back door soaked in perspiration and smelling of fresh-cut grass. He joins Hugh for lunch, sitting cross-legged on the floor next to the recliner while Krista and I run out to pick up flowers and cake at the store.

Hugh's parents arrive as we prepare a quick summer dinner of southern fried chicken, salads, and ice cream. The afternoon and evening begins to feel like a holiday. Krista entertains the girls with stories about the time she danced in her high school production of *Cinderella* and spends the night with us before the big day of the recital.

Sunday becomes an actual day of rest so Hugh will be awake for the show at night. After relaxing all day, our entourage heads to the theatre in three cars. I hold tight to Hugh's leather woven belt that doubles as his gait belt while we walk from the parking deck to the Mosque. He has refused to wear his helmet and ball cap. I hold his belt sturdily as we rush to make it to the head of the line that is building up outside so we can find our saved seats before the doors to the house open. We are a few minutes too slow. Just as we approach the entrance, the doors swing open and throngs of people pour into the theater. Hugh, minding his impeccable manners, holds the door for everyone and will not budge. Frozen in his role as doorman, he smiles as one person after another nods "thank you" to him. I stand just ahead of him, motioning with my hand. "Hugh, come on in. Everyone's waiting. We need to get our seats."

"You are so rude," he mouths to me as he continues to let grateful patron after grateful patron squish through the doors, nodding pleasantly at every one.

In an effort to encourage Hugh to enter the building, his father decides to hold the door next to him, thinking Hugh will let go of his door. It doesn't work. In fact, Hugh probably thinks his father is following his lead and is proud of his manners. Both men now hold the two heavy theater doors open for the entire crowd, and together, they let over 100 people into the building. Hugh's father glances nervously at his son. Hugh doesn't budge. Up ahead, his mother leans on her cane watching us. She gives me a "what can we do" shrug. We exchange worried looks. When my eyebrows shoot up in surrender, we both break out laughing.

Finally, Hugh decides to enter the lobby. His father stays close to him until I can grab his belt. As I walk next to his father, I whisper, "What did you do to that boy when he was little—*beat* those manners into him?" He smiles down at me and elbows me in the ribs.

As we swarm with the crowd to the designated area where we are told seats are being held for us, we see a Shuffles employee throwing her body over the seats and defending them from an elderly man who claims they are his seats. My arm becomes an instant field of goose bumps as blasts of air-conditioning blow on us. Hugh zips his sweatshirt all the way up and settles into his springboard folding seat. The recital will be about three hours long and very loud, so our plan is to have Jim pick Hugh up out front during intermission and whisk him home. When the girls arrive home after the show, Hugh will surprise them with bouquets of flowers.

As the music starts I hand Hugh the foam earplugs so the high volume won't give him a headache. He slowly takes them from my hands and looks down with a quizzical expression, then puts the earplugs in his mouth and with an awful scrunched-up face says, "What is this?" I pull on his arm when I see him chewing the earplugs. "They are *earplugs*, not marshmallows. Take them out of your mouth!" He spits them out and stuffs the damp buds in his ears, laughing. Finally the curtain comes up and I sink into my seat. Hugh and I beam with pride watching Mary and Anna perform.

About thirty minutes into the show, Hugh leans toward me and says, "I have to GO. Now!" The theater is cavernous and the bathroom is far away upstairs.

"Dad, can you get him to the men's room? I don't think they'll let me in!" I whisper. The trip takes a long time. Afterward, his father says that Hugh insisted on using every paper towel in the dispenser. His behavior was becoming more erratic as he tired.

At intermission, I help Hugh down the long wide ramp into the ornate lobby and through the glass doors to the sidewalk. Jim has managed to park right at the curb, exactly in front of us. "You'd make a great New York cabbie," I tell him. Hugh eagerly gets in the car.

"Ready to watch the NBA game?" Jim asks. Hugh nods and blows me a kiss. I wave as they pull away to the sound of music building for the second act.

Krista scoots over to fill Hugh's empty seat. After the final curtain, she says her good-byes on the street. Electra treats the girls to a ride home in her sports car while I drive Hugh's parents back to the house.

Inside, Hugh is waiting expectantly with two thick bouquets for his daughters to kick off the after-party. Anna and Mary's friends stream in behind us and congregate around the kitchen snacking and laughing. Hugh claims his recliner, and before long, his head tips to the side as he dozes off, oblivious to the noise surrounding him. "I'm so glad Dad got to see us dance," Mary says kissing my cheek.

At the end of this gala event, I hear Hugh's father say, "I'll get that." I catch his eye and smirk in jest as he rushes to hold the front door for two girls on their way out.

Chapter 25

Mrs. Rawlins,

*You and your family are very strong. Before you know it, Mr. Rawlins will be
back mowing the grass and doing the chores. Until then, I'm here if you need me.
Just remember, he's Huperman after all!*

Love,

Christie

- Anna's best friend

Eight-ten weeks out

D r. G looks up from his notes. "Hugh is exhibiting insight, which
is rare in individuals with Hugh's severity of injury," he says.
He's referring to Hugh's ability to perceive that he has a problem, and
that he is frustrated at not being able to achieve results more quickly.
He says it's a good sign from a recovery point of view.

Nancy approaches the subject of "letting go" during one of my
private counseling sessions. I am having trouble knowing what Hugh
should and should not be doing on his own. Due to balance issues
and the soft spot on his skull, my inclination is to stick close to him.
"I know I often do things for him because he's slow and I'm tired of
everything taking so long," I tell her.

"You're right, that's no help to him. Try to wait longer for him to
accomplish a task without jumping in," she suggests. "It will pay off in
the long run."

Containing my nervous energy has become impossible. I often feel like I'm ready to bolt. I begin cleaning when I feel antsy instead of fussing over Hugh. Cleaning is therapy for me—a mess that can be easily wiped up or straightened out. The results are easily observable: order out of chaos, beauty out of grime. People begin to comment at how neat my house is all the time. "With all you have to do…how do you keep up with it?" I hear. They don't know this tidy space represents a fragile island of perfection on the outside that masks the unfixable mess I feel inside.

One hot night after a walk and a shower, Hugh lies on the bed wrapped in a towel. He's beginning to drift off to sleep when I ask, "Ready to put some pajamas on?" He slowly opens his eyes, picks up the television remote, points it at me, and clicks. "You do know you *cannot* turn me off with that thing!" I say in an exasperated voice.

Continuing to click, he responds, "At least I can turn down the volume or change the channel!" A smile creeps across his face. Giving in, I flop next to him and wiggle the remote out of the way. "Okay, so sleep in your towel, but take your pills."

The next night, Hugh's old bike racing teammates, Greg Florence and Larry Piper, come over. Larry is trying to figure out if Hugh will need any legal help down the road and wants to hear the details of Hugh's injury. When I tell them that Hugh never went through the cursing/ throwing stuff stage, Hugh throws a grape at my head and pipes up, "Hey, what do you mean!" This new clownish side of him catches me off guard.

"Very funny. Stop," I say. Hugh lobs another grape and hits my forehead. Everyone laughs but me. "Hugh, can we listen to what Larry has to say?" I ask. His smirk says I'm a killjoy. Larry pulls out some papers and asks us a few questions, but when we tell him we have Liz on the case, he says he may just want to review the medical evaluations Hugh gets for court to be sure we include everything.

As the school year winds down, the girls seem to need a ride somewhere every night. Dinners are swallowed whole, on our feet. Schedules are so tight, I never see my friends. When Electra calls I rush her off the phone. "Wait!" she says before hanging up. "You are scheduled for a massage, June 13th at ten o'clock. Be there!" I gladly obey.

Lying on the draped table at Therapeutic Arts, I smell the lavender candle and bask in the soothing instrumental music as Electra pinches, pushes, and kneads the knots out of my tense body. As she finishes up, she says, "That was like massaging a brick. I think you need to come in every week!"

"Now *this* is what our insurance *should* cover," I say, looking a bit drunk from the headiness of her pampering.

The girls finish their last day of the IB Middle Years program on June 14th. The date completely sneaks up on me. I've been absent from their lives. It seems like there should be more of a celebration in our usual style. Instead, it's just another day void of plans or any air of excitement other than recognition in a school assembly. They've both achieved honor roll all three years. At breakfast, I apologize for not even having a greeting card for them. They shrug it off. "Oh, it's no big deal, Mom," Anna says. "Nothing special," Mary agrees. I promise them I will be the first to stand up and cheer at the assembly, a bit of my old enthusiasm leaking out. "No!" screams Anna, laughing. "Mom, no standing ovation! Promise?" Mary chimes in.

"Okay, how about right now?" I stand at the breakfast table in my pajamas and applaud. The girls run around the table and give me a hug.

At the assembly, I think about how Anna and Mary pulled off stellar grades this final year in middle school in spite of their tumultuous home life. I sit in awe of them and brim over with love knowing what they have achieved in the midst of so much family drama. Bambi is next to me, shooting digital pictures of Harley and the girls to mark the occasion, but my joy is diluted by Hugh's absence. He is struggling to complete simple word problems in therapy at the same moment that Mary and Anna accept certificates for honor roll.

That night, the girls go out to an end-of-the-year party at a friend's house, and I rent the movie *Vanilla Sky* to watch with Hugh, knowing nothing in advance about the film. It is a long, involved story with elements of a car crash, injury, and amnesia. I just can't believe my poor timing. Hugh seems oblivious to the storyline. He is reclining in his Lay-Z-Boy. I am lying on the couch, my head propped by a throw pillow. All of a sudden, my cell phone rings in my pocketbook on the rocking chair across from me. Since it's after nine-thirty, I bolt up thinking something must be wrong with the girls.

I hear Hugh's low voice. "Hi hon. I'm thinking of you."

I swing my head around to see him smiling in the recliner on his cell phone. Instinctively I walk into the dining room, away from him, and continue to talk into my phone.

"I'm right here," I say tenderly. "Don't you like the movie?"

"It's okay," he says softly.

"Why did you call me? We're in the same room." The call feels intimate, fun.

"I was just thinking about you so I thought I'd call you and tell you."

"That is very sweet," I say, smiling into a cell phone that suddenly feels like a precious possession. We talk about nothing awhile, holding through silences, not wanting to hang up. For the rest of the evening, until the girls come home around midnight, we watch each other more than the movie. I stare at him in disbelief that he's here. He stares at me as if trying to get to know me all over again.

The first week of summer break is busy and noisy at the house with the girls home all day. They decide to forego swim team since they both have summer trips planned, but they have signed up for a tap class at Shuffles. Summer will be different this year—Hugh will be home often during the day and he needs quiet rest. This limits our once noisy sleepover house and the amount of time I can spend shuttling the girls to activities.

As for the general atmosphere, Anna and Mary overhear me on the phone with doctors, insurance companies, and therapists all day long. Our house takes on a serious tone, not much like the usual breezy summer months of old. Mary and Anna work hard not to add to the workload or ask for too much. During the hours that Hugh is at rehab, I try to complete some office work when I'm not driving the girls to the pool or to a friend's house. I need to be home when he returns.

Hugh is obsessed with two things later in June: his cell phone and buying a car. He wants to take his cell phone with him to rehab but it's not permitted. He sneaks it anyway one day and calls his office. When caught, he's told to promptly put it away. He tells me people treat him like a child. But it's not being able to drive that really upsets him, and it bothers him that we no longer own two cars. He asks constantly if we can go to the dealership to look at cars on the market. Unfortunately, buying cars is at the top of the list of things I hate to do most, and I really can't see the point of looking when Hugh is not permitted to drive. It is a source of tension between us, another example of how his independence has been cut off.

Upon leaving rehab at MCV, Hugh was told he was not to drive until he was given the medical "go ahead." One thing everyone would be on the lookout for was seizures. He has had none so far. The other problem is cognitive speed, his processing and reaction time. Driving is a complex and inherently dangerous activity that requires the driver to scan, assess, and respond quickly and safely.

When hearing Hugh's nostalgic voice as he talks about driving, you would think the loss of his driving privilege was the saddest consequence of his injury. He is relentless in asking, "When can I drive again?" He wants his independence and freedom back. I hide the car keys, thinking fondly how his "no rules" motto has helped him develop capable managers at work. He often tells people, "I'd rather you ask forgiveness than permission." This is his way of entrusting his staff with decision-making power, and letting people learn from their own mistakes without fear of retribution.

On a warm June afternoon, he suggests again, "Hey, let's look at cars!" as if he hasn't asked and been turned down a million times before. I can no longer think of reasons not to take him. It's more tiring to continually deny him, so I agree to go.

"I don't want that helmet," he says scratching his head.

"Okay, it's hot," I say, deciding to be extra vigilant with him. "But stop scratching or you'll bleed."

"Stop telling me what to do," he says. I jam my thumbnail in my mouth. "And don't bite your nails!" he adds, looking smug, now that he has something to nag me about. My cuticle bleeds. "See, now you're bleeding!" he says, extra pleased.

"Dear God, we're a pair," I say.

As we enter the showroom, the salesman avoids looking at Hugh, speaking only to me. Hugh's head is sunken in. His eyes and expression look robotic. I can see that the salesman knows there is something wrong with Hugh and doesn't want to stare, so he ignores him, talks past him, and avoids eye contact. Even when Hugh asks the salesman a direct question, the salesman looks at me with the answer. Hugh is wearing his woven leather belt, an improvised method I sometimes substitute for the gait belt. By now, I am used to keeping my hand on the back of this belt all the time as a matter of habit; in fact, I've recently developed tennis elbow from holding on to him all day long. I try to imagine the salesman's assumptions from his expression of pity and repugnance, but I don't offer any explanations. His demeanor bugs me.

"We're only browsing," I say casually. "Mind if we just walk the lot?" The salesman looks relieved to not have to deal with us. He's free to *neglect* us. I think about the word.

"Neglect" is a TBI word. It's one of the hardest symptoms of TBI for me to understand. I was told Hugh has left neglect. He no longer notices things on his left side, including the left-sided parts of his body. He has trouble reading words on the left side of a page. If he is filling out a form, he sometimes leaves the left side blank and only completes the right side. He does not look to his left or see things on his left. This is a dangerous situation when he is out walking—and it must be improved if he's to drive. His occupational therapist works with him daily to see that he compensates for this tendency by reinforcing habits to always check left, in the hope that it becomes second nature to him at some point.

Today, neglect causes him to constantly bang into the rearview mirrors on his left side as we walk through the narrow rows of cars. Hugh's left elbow is still raw and oozing from a deep wound he sustained in the crash. It is made worse by his banging it into things. By the time we leave the car lot, it is sore and bleeding. We are both dissatisfied with the outing. I lack enthusiasm, and he is totally frustrated because he's not allowed to test-drive any cars. As we finish up our grumpy stroll on the black pavement, I feel guilty for not being more pleasant on the excursion, so I suggest we treat ourselves to a Dairy Queen. Pulling out of the parking lot, I run over the curb, jarring Hugh so that his ice cream plops on his shirt. The look he shoots me says it all: "I can't wait till I can drive and I will drive better than that!"

After months of having driving help, I am reluctant to bother people with constant requests, but managing the driving schedule for a busy family of four is grating on my nerves. Occasionally, our friends still fill in the blanks. Bambi registers Harley for tap classes with the girls and graciously offers to drive the group nearly every week. It is a relief not to have to ask. I am quickly becoming the friend nobody wants anymore. Even if I don't ask for a favor, everyone knows I probably need one at any given moment, and that makes me cringe. Little by little, our friends have naturally drifted back to their own busy lives and we are more on our own.

We have a follow-up appointment to see a doctor from the MCV Rehab Center. I insist I can do the trip alone with Hugh, even though his father has offered to help. Admittedly, I can be as obstinate as my husband. "Besides," I tell him, "they have valet parking." His dad is now a constant presence at our house. He's taken over lawn duty from Hugh's friends and has reorganized the garage. He tries to cover all the bases and take care of things he thinks Hugh might have done.

Once downtown, I see that valet parking is full. Now we have to park in the eight-floor parking garage at MCV nearby. The parking deck elevator we ride to street level smells ripe with sweat and feels like a greenhouse. Rivers of water run down the sides of Hugh's face from under his helmet while I steady him with the gait belt. We step out the elevator door and both inhale deeply as if finding oxygen after a dive, then we walk a few city blocks to the medical building. Outside, the one hundred degree air bloats my hair with humidity. A thin film of sweat coats my skin. It's afternoon, Hugh's tired time. He's usually napping by now after a hard morning at rehab. "C'mon Hon, a few more steps," I cajole. "We're almost there."

After seeing a medical student for twenty minutes, we wait an hour to see the doctor. As time drags on, I grow anxious about getting Hugh safely back to the parking deck, down the elevator and into the car. He looks more tired by the second, slumped in the waiting room chair, his long legs stretched so far out in front of him that a toddler trips over them.

At last we are called in. This doctor has never met Hugh before, but in a clinical voice, he tells me that Hugh should have made his most significant gains in the first few months and from here on out, progress will slow down. *Slow down,* I think. *How much slower can it get?* This man's detached assessment feels like an insulting dismissal. Hugh is improving every day and he is not yet near where I feel he will go. We've been given all kinds of markers for recovery: three months, six months, a year, or more. What are we supposed to believe? While tying ourselves down to deadlines is futile, we want a little optimism!

I sit in a cold metal chair watching my husband go through the same examination I've seen ten times before. I want answers. As I watch the doctor talking to his clipboard in his doctorly way, I hear echoes of Dr. Ward's advice: *ignore the dates. Hugh will continue to improve. Just go about life.*

I manage to get Hugh back to the car while he leans heavily on me, but it takes every ounce of my strength to hold onto his gait belt. When we arrive home and he is planted safely in his chair, I feel the bad news weigh on me. I want to sleep or shower; I'm drenched in sweat, but it's dinnertime. The girls are bored. "Can you drive us to the movies tonight?" Mary asks with an eager face. "We're tired of always asking friends for a ride."

"We'll see," I say mindlessly as I start assembling a salad, but they know the answer is no.

At our next team meeting, Hugh's PT, Jennifer, reports that he's beginning to run on a treadmill, very slowly. He still has left foot drop and drags that foot sometimes when he walks, especially when he's tired. Hugh tells me about running on the treadmill in front of a full-length mirror so he can see his own movements and concentrate on them. "I have to tell myself to bend my knee, lift my toes, while watching the movement," he says. "Just lifting my foot higher requires a huge mental effort." I try to imagine what this is like for him, but I can't really relate to it in my own experience.

Penny reports that she is working on his upper extremities with him. His left shoulder is frozen and he has trouble lifting his arm. His forearm, wrist, hands, and fingers are all affected. They hang limp, moving slightly only when Hugh concentrates hard. It will take time to build new pathways.

Michaelle, his speech therapist, reports that his motor cortex is

affected, so it's difficult to plan, initiate, and create the movement necessary to follow through on his left side. She has him do "smiling" exercises
to keep the muscles on the left side of his face in working order until he
builds new pathways. Hugh's smile now looks crooked and unbalanced.
This symptom falls under the huge umbrella of his left neglect. I tell him
it makes him look like Harrison Ford. Michaelle ends her report with
encouraging news: "His memory is showing marked improvement."

The tone of the meeting is upbeat, honest, and somewhat positive. Each team member is obviously interested in Hugh's physical,
emotional, psychological, and cognitive health. Of course, the meeting
ends with a question from Hugh.

"When do you think I'll be able to drive?"

Everyone looks at the floor.

Chapter 26

June 26, 2002
I really wish I could make all your problems disappear. Hang in there. Keep en-
couraging Hugh – we all know he can do it! I am going to miss you this week.
Love,
Susan

-Susan Healey, sister-in-law

Ten – eleven weeks out

We struggle with the decision of whether to cancel our vacation with family to celebrate the fiftieth anniversary of my parents' wedding in St. Augustine, Florida. Both Dr. Ward and Dr. G. tell me it's possible, but not necessarily advisable. I'm advised that if we go, I should find a local doctor just in case and make sure that Hugh stays out of the waves. Considering how much he loves the ocean, this is not welcome news. The thought of flying with the pressure in his head is worrisome too, but driving could be worse. He often gets carsick. "What is your gut feeling about going?" I ask Hugh as we walk around the block.

He pauses and says, "Not to go. I want to, but I don't think we should." We decide we will stay home, but I make plans for the girls to go.

The decision leaves me feeling cheated and sad for days. All my five brothers and sisters live out of state and I desperately need a dose of their wild Irish humor. The bright spot is that Anna and Mary will have a real vacation, and if I'm honest with myself, they will have a much better time if they get a break from us right now.

Kate and her two daughters arrive to pick up the girls; my parents pull in around the same time. They plan to spend two nights with us before driving south to Florida. I realize our decision to stay behind is the right one when I see how this small group of loud, excited relatives tires Hugh out. It doesn't help that Hugh and I feel separated by circumstances from the family's party mood.

Between walks around the block and mealtimes, Kate patiently works with Hugh on his home exercises from rehab. She stretches his left arm and leg, remarking that his left side has grown weaker. His left arm and hand are nearly useless. He wears a brace to hold his wrist up, otherwise it hangs limp. He can barely move his fingers at all. Rehab prescribes wall push-ups at home. I place his left hand on the wall next to his right hand, only to watch it slide down during the first push up. I keep replacing it on the wall. Hugh's face falls each time his hand slides down and I can see he is anxious to lie in bed and sleep it off. When Kate is around, he tries harder and keeps going. "One more push-up, then I'll rest," he says.

"That's the spirit!" she encourages.

Every time I pass Hugh in his chair, I stretch his arm. "The poor guy! Is that really necessary all the time?" my mother asks.

"Yes, it is. If I keep his range of motion up, he will use it again someday." She looks at me with sad eyes. "Rosemary, can't you ever relax?"

"No, Mom, I guess I can't. If I relax I may think. And if I think, I'll have questions like 'Why did this have to happen?' Questions with no answers. If I sit down to relax, I'm afraid I won't get back up again." She nods in understanding. An expression crosses her face, one of concern that her oldest daughter is dangerously stressed. Her blue eyes crease. I imagine her saying a silent prayer for me, and feel a sting of regret for snapping at her.

"Sorry, Mom. We need to get to the doctor by eleven," I say, helping Hugh out of his chair. Kate accompanies us to the follow-up surgical appointment with Dr. Ward. He checks Hugh's head where the piece of skull was removed and decides the swelling has receded far enough. Again, we discuss the emotional side of these past few months. Dr. Ward expresses his dislike for the strict helmet rules and what they represent to his patients: fear. "In my twenty-plus years as a neurosurgeon," he says, "I have never seen a patient fall and re-injure his compression site, and yet patients are made to feel vulnerable until their bone flap is replaced."

Dr. Ward always stresses quality-of-life issues for patients and their families. His direct and practical nature reminds me so much of the pre-injury Hugh that I strongly connect with him. When he tests Hugh's left arm, he says there is still a significant loss of tone. He was hoping for much more improvement.

Hugh appears timid on this visit. "When can you fix my divot?" he asks.

The doctor grins and says, "How about three weeks from now?" Looking at a calendar, he adds, "Let's say, July 23rd."

"Will I be knocked out?" Hugh asks.

"Don't worry, you won't feel or remember a thing. That's all you need to know. This is an easy, routine surgery, nothing to be afraid of."

I mention that we were told that Hugh has pretty much healed as much as he will and that progress will slow down. "What do you think?" I ask.

I read disappointment on his face mixed with a bit of annoyance. "It's only been a few months. I like to use six months or a year as an indicator of turnout for a patient. The brain takes time to heal, and there are vast differences in each person's case. After a year, progress may slow down, but it *will continue* for up to two years or more," he says.

Dr. Ward says that there is now data to suggest that the brain continues to recover indefinitely, and that this whole area of study is still new, so really, we might find there is subtle lifelong improvement. "It's hard to measure or determine if the patient's brain is healing or if compensatory strategies are working. But what does it matter?" he states, palms up. "So long as the patient can get back to living, the result is what counts."

Results. This doctor speaks Hugh's language. I see a spark of hope.

While we are visiting Dr. Ward, the cousins are at home baking a three-tiered anniversary cake for their grandparents. My cell phone rings and it's Mary. "Mom, the cake has collapsed," she says. I can hear her sister and two cousins laughing in the background. "We need more pink frosting to patch it up. Can you pick some up on your way home? It's a surprise for Nan and Pop." The afternoon flies by with walks, drinks, and a sit down dinner.

"Check out the leaning tower of wedding cake," Anna whispers to me later. We all sing "Happy Anniversary to You" for Mom and Pop. While I watch the cake cutting ceremony, Dr. Ward's philosophy comes to mind: *Who cares if it's slightly lopsided as long as it's delicious?*

Chapter 27

I want to send you another note of congratulations on tomorrow's celebration of just short of a quarter century of having a life together, filled as life is with fun, love, worries, a lot of little ones, and even a biggish one once in a long while... But holy socks, you've had nothing but big days all of this past week, so rejoice and keep looking up to the stars as Dante really would have said. Right on, you two, Love and everything else,
Azever,
Link

-Hugh's uncle, O. Lincoln Igou, New Paltz, NY

Eleven-twelve weeks out

Our week without the girls passes quickly. On July 1st, our actual twenty-fourth wedding anniversary, Hugh has rehab, so I meet him in the courtyard for lunch. At night, we join Hugh's parents at their home for dinner. His mother nudges me on my way out the door. "It was great the way he talked about the stock market," she says smiling.

"I know. He is starting to watch the news sometimes too," I tell her. At home, the girls call from St. Augustine to wish us Happy Anniversary and fight for the phone to tell us the big news of the day: "Uncle Danny's bathing suit came down while he was boogie boarding."

The rest of our week is full with visits from friends. Fred, the manager of the bike store that Hugh frequents, comes by to surprise Hugh with a new, sleek Giro helmet, like the ones in the Tour de France. In the late afternoon on Wednesday, the CFO of Hugh's company swings by for a visit. I wince when Hugh greets him by asking, "So how do you like my divot?" as he points to the dent in his head. Unfazed, Brett takes Hugh for a spin in his convertible Porsche, a major thrill ride. He tells Hugh he purchased it on e-Bay. I see Hugh's mind churning: Note to self: buy Porsche 911 on Internet when I can drive.

That evening, Jim comes over for dinner. I indulge in two glasses of merlot and it makes me giddy. We all saunter out for a walk. Hugh is stumbling, I am weaving, and Jim is guiding. "I don't know which one to hold tighter," Jim says. After a lap around the block, he shepherds us through the front door, up the stairs and watches us flop onto the bed before leaving. "Sweet dreams you two."

"Night, Jim," I say as he shows himself out of our house and locks the door.

Thursday is Independence Day. We sleep in, and by the time we wake up, it is already in the high eighties outside. "Let's walk to Kinko's," Hugh says. He has set a goal to walk a full mile, all the way to Broad Street through the subdivision of Lexington, a walking route we used to take all the time. At the halfway point I've already had enough. "Want to turn around?" I ask. Sweat pours in rivers down his face from under his thick helmet.

"No, keep going," he puffs. His eyes appear more lucid, pierced with determination. He is going to go the limit if it kills him. I hold tight to his gait belt. Nearing the end of the walk, we stop in the shade a few times, and I offer to flag a car. He refuses. I'm cursing myself for not bringing a water bottle. We are both drenched and my elbow radiates pain from holding the gait belt steady. Hugh is ornery, hot, and tired. But the second we arrive home, he flops into his recliner and shouts, "We made it!"

Flipping on the television, we hear a heat advisory; our local TV station is warning the elderly and infirm to stay indoors for record-breaking temperatures of over one hundred. We clink our iced tea glasses together in sweet victory. "We made it in one hundred degrees!" Hugh cheers.

Near the end of the week, while Hugh's parents are over, Hugh walks from the kitchen to the living room, catches his left foot on the rug, and launches toward the pointed edge of the fireplace mantel. He's without his helmet. Rita lets out a scream. I lurch forward, but I'm too far away to help. My nerves tingle. Hugh's right hand shoots out and he catches himself before falling. "I'm okay, Mom," he yells with his Harrison Ford smile. Rita is clutching her chest.

"I cannot wait for that bone to be replaced!" I say. "Wish I could roll you in bubble wrap!"

At the end of the week, my parents and Kate return home with the kids bearing gifts and videos of the week's events. Mary holds the T-shirt up to Hugh's chest to see if it's a good fit. "Like it, Dad?" she asks. "Matches your eyes!"

"I like anything you give me, honey," he says, kissing the top of her head. "I missed you. And you!" he adds, kissing Anna's head too.

Anna holds out two small gift bags for me. "And for Mom...," she says, proudly. A square candle in a black metal holder is wrapped in paper. The other bag contains a watercolor of St. George Street in St. Augustine, painted by a local artist. "What a thoughtful gift. I love the colors in this!" I say, wishing I could have walked that street with them.

Hugh tires quickly again with all the noise and confusion around luggage, stomping up and down stairs, and general merriment. He retreats upstairs after a short while. An hour or two later, we all join him on the big bed in the guest room to watch home movies taken during the past week. Clips of the anniversary toast, a shared family meal, chicken fights in the pool, boogie boarding and surfing lead to many funny stories. Close-ups of happy sunburned faces fill in the summer scenery. In these moving images, I can smell the salt air. A deep melancholy aches in my chest as I watch our daughters with family, having so much fun. *Will we ever have fun again?* As if he heard my thoughts, Hugh locks his fingers in mine.

Chapter 28

Anna writes in my journal:
I asked Dad if he was nervous about his surgery and he said, "Yes" so I asked,
"Why?" He said, "I'm not afraid of dying. I just don't want to be away from you,
Mary and your Mama."

Thirteen –fourteen weeks out

I decide to talk to Penny about Hugh's left arm that seems worse lately. It is permanently bent at the elbow as if he's wearing an invisible sling across his chest. I meet her at HealthSouth during one of Hugh's therapy visits.

"It takes all my strength to straighten his arm, it's so rigid. What's happening?" I ask her.

"I've noticed it too," she says.

"I've been stretching it several times a day. Anna and Mary help him stretch too, but he can't straighten it on his own and his left hand is so weak he can't hold a cup, a pencil, or even lift his wrist without immense effort. I'm beginning to think he may not regain the use of that arm."

"I know it seems worse, but actually his contractions signify the return of messages transmitted by the brain. I think he'll regain the use of his arm and hand eventually. Sometimes, when the brain begins sending and receiving those messages again, they are just not quite right at first—either too strong or a bit misdirected. But the fact that he is having strong reactions in his arm is a good thing. It can indicate neurological healing." I leave feeling better and hope she's right.

Hugh is switched from everyday therapy to three times a week. On his days off, I take on the task of helping him with cognitive assignments to save visits. Sitting at the kitchen table together, I ask him to find today's weather report and let me know what to expect. Hugh slowly scans the paper. After several minutes, he still can't locate it. I suggest he check the front page to see where the weather page is. "B6, Metro section," he says. Now he sifts through the stack of papers to find the Metro section. With eyebrows knitted in concentration, he reads today's forecast aloud. Setting the paper down, he stares at my face, smiling. These private proud moments bind us, these inches of achievement.

The next morning Hugh has therapy at HealthSouth. Our insurance only covers sixty therapy visits per year, and we are using them up fast. Once those sixty are used, the cost will be completely out-of-pocket. I am busy with résumé writing work. I have two jobs to complete and a delivery to make. I finish writing at the computer in my office and take Mary to the bank and CVS to buy items for her impending school trip to Spain. We rush home in time to meet Hugh's taxi and fix him some lunch. He is due home at 12:15. After unpacking Mary's items and assembling a turkey sandwich for Hugh, I wait in my office.

It is not too unusual for cabs to be a little late, but by one o'clock, he still has not shown up. Up the street at Starbucks, a client is waiting for me to deliver his résumé. I call HealthSouth to find out where Hugh might be. The transportation message machine picks up, so I ask them to check on Hugh's cab and call me, then tell Mary to wait and call my cell phone the minute he gets in. The fear in her face is palpable; I suggest that maybe they are held up by a new patient in a wheel chair. Hating to leave, I pull away to deliver my résumé quickly, checking in with Mary once by phone to find that Hugh is still not home. Where is that taxi? At one-thirty Mary calls in a panic; she's crying on the phone as I turn into the neighborhood. "There's a man coming to the house, Mom, I don't know who it is. I never saw the car before, but it's not a taxi."

"Stay inside, Mary, I'll be right home." I race the car around the corner and see at once that it's our dentist's car. He has come to mow the lawn again. Beside herself with fear and crying uncontrollably, Mary is too embarrassed to answer the door when he knocks. I rush over, open the door, and explain what's going on to Dr. Norris.

"Hugh's really late from rehab," I tell him. "Mary didn't recognize your car; she was expecting a taxi and it scared her. She thought it might be a representative from HealthSouth sent to deliver bad news about her father." As I say the words, I realize how fragile our world has become; we expect disaster to lurk around every corner.

"I'm sure it's nothing, just a delay of some sort," Dr. Norris says. He walks to the garage for the mower with an air of calm that helps us settle down a bit. After calling the transportation department again, I sit on the front stoop with Mary. Finally, at one-forty, the phone rings. The cab has been lost. It is a new, young driver and Hugh had trouble giving him directions. Holding my hand over the phone, I tell Mary he's okay. We both exhale. When I explain to her what happened, she's angry with the driver. "Why didn't he call us?"

"I guess he's new on the job and didn't want to get in trouble." I say. She stares at me. "Maybe he thought he wasn't that late." Mary throws me a look of disgust. I mimic her anger, "Maybe he's a stupid idiot? A moron? A dope? A jack…" I offer.

"Mom!" she laughs, as the taxi arrives. Hugh is nauseated from the long drive and heat, compounded by the fact that he is dressed in sweats and has a pounding headache. We're exhausted from worry, but relieved to see him home. Deep-set shadows under his eyes give him a sunken look. "My stomach hurts," he moans, carsick. We help him to his recliner and Mary hands him a cold glass of water. I can see he wants to sleep, but his queasiness keeps him tossing in the chair.

An hour later, my sister Kate calls and Hugh answers. He tells her he had a great time in Florida before he hands me the phone.

"Hey Roe, Hugh talked about Florida like he was there. Is he okay?" she asks. "I didn't know what to tell him. I didn't want to say he wasn't there."

"Kate, he's had an awful day. His cab got lost and he was over-heated and carsick. He's really overtired and confused."

"Maybe because of the video he saw of all of us on the beach?" she suggests.

"Could be, or a dream, or just that he's so overtired now. I don't know."

After we hang up, I sit on Hugh's lap in the recliner, my arms around his neck. "You were talking to Kate about the beach trip to St. Augustine. Do you remember that you and I stayed home? Only the girls went."

Hugh looks puzzled and worried. He furrows his eyebrows. "But I remember the waves and rubbing sunscreen on your back," he says.

"It might have been an older memory or the video we saw. We didn't go there." A look of sadness crosses his face. I feel like I'm taking something precious away from him. "You might have thought about it a lot or had a really good dream about it. We never went there, honey." Hugh leans back, thinking for a minute, then slowly closes his eyes as I continue, "It's okay. Sometimes it seems like we did things when you hear about them so much. That's all. Try and get some sleep."

As I watch him doze off, I secretly wish I could jump inside his version of reality. I need a vacation badly.

Over dinner, I notice Hugh pocketing again. He chews up his food and stores it in his left cheek, leaving it there. He doesn't realize it's there—another peculiar part of his left neglect. After a time, he makes an awful face and spits out the food as if wondering how in the world it got there. When I see his cheek puff out again, I remind him. "Food in your cheek, Hon. Remember what the therapist said." He puts his right pointer finger in his mouth and swipes the food to the center so he can swallow.

"I want to lie down. I'm really tired," he says after eating. I walk him over to his recliner and go upstairs to check on Mary. Her school trip to Spain is fast approaching. It's taken a back seat to everything else going on, so we've barely had time to prepare. I find her packing a suitcase with a serious look on her face. Clothes are strewn all over the bed with a neatly penned checklist of items she wants to bring along.

"Hey, how's it going? You don't look too excited." I say.

"Oh, I am. I just hate leaving home right now with Dad's operation and all," she says. While she's in Spain, Hugh will have his final surgery. She and her father are scheduled to come home on the same day, she from Spain, and he from the hospital.

"Dad wants you to go on this trip," I tell her. "You've been planning this trip for two years and it's the only big trip you'll have before college. Plus, you'll see him the very first day after his surgery.

Mary perks up, but then looks down at the carpet. "I know Mom," she says. "I just feel bad that you'll all be at the hospital again."

"We'll be fine. Mary, if anyone deserves a little fun, it's you. Go and have a great time. Dr. Ward said this operation is much easier. Dad'll be fine." She hugs me and manages a weak smile of resignation.

"I love you, Mom. I'm going to miss you," she says.

"No you won't. You'll be way too busy to even think about us, and that's the way it should be. Besides, we'll talk on the phone. Now finish packing!" I leave her in a much happier mood and run down the stairs feeling better.

Sitting in his recliner across from the banister in the family room, Hugh stares in wonder as I rush down the steps. "You run up and down those stairs so easily, sometimes it makes me jealous. You're such an inspiration to me."

I laugh. "Wow, that's a role reversal!" I say. "You'll be doing the same thing soon, I'm sure."

Hugh has several pre-op appointments scheduled during the week, and between his impending surgery and Mary's trip, our front door swings open hourly. Talk of surgery and the hospital disturbs Hugh. He is not looking forward to it. On Sunday, July 14th, Electra brings over a box of bagels for breakfast. Always the therapist, she can't resist working on Hugh's arm. While she chats with us, she pushes and pulls his left arm in all directions. Hugh is unmotivated to stretch on his own, but minding his manners, he cooperates with his favorite masseuse.

Later, Hugh's administrative assistant from work, Michelle, drops by with her family to wish him luck. In the evening, Mary's friend, Amanda, joins us for a Bon Voyage dinner to say goodbye to Mary. Hugh looks weepy at the thought of her leaving.

By Monday, I have a lot of trouble getting Hugh out of bed. When he finally stands up, he falls hard into the green dressing table, banging his hip on the way down. A deep purple bruise forms immediately. I run downstairs, grab a bag of frozen peas, and put it on the bruise. "That's too cold!" he says.

"You always used to use ice on your back," I say. "You used to tell me a bruise would go away quicker if you iced it right away, remember?"

"Oh yeah," he says with a shiver. "Give me another blanket, though."

Hugh is clearly backsliding, totally unfocused, and I don't know why. I begin to wonder if he has reached a plateau. We've been told this will happen periodically. It is agony waiting out a plateau because we never know if it will end. One day the progress will stop and that will be when we know the true extent of his injury.

I try to imagine Hugh's perspective. Tensions are mounting: the upcoming traffic court hearing for the woman who hit him, his newfound insight about his condition, and his impending surgery. This afternoon Mary leaves for Spain. Separation from the girls is hard on him. His new sentimental side is puppy-doggish. He's a man infatuated with his children, thriving on their affection. Tears well up at the mention of an old baby memory, surprising even him.

When the three of us go to see Mary off, it's a hot humid day, so Hugh has trouble standing in the parking lot with twenty-four excited teenagers and their doting parents dwarfed by the large bus. He keeps stumbling and almost falls over. "It's too hot out here, let's wait in the car," I suggest. We sit in the Explorer with the air conditioner running while Mary runs back and forth, kissing us and loading her luggage. In a way it's heartbreaking—all I want to do is bolt from the car and go hug her, but then I see her run off holding hands with Anna and realize how tightly connected they've become by navigating this difficult time together. In the parking lot, they hug for an extra long time before they break away laughing at some shared secret.

Mary runs over to the window of the Explorer one last time before leaving. Hugh rolls it down and says some fatherly things to her. His questions are suited to a kindergartener. "Can you remember my cell phone number in case you need to call me?" Dutifully, she recites every number, looking straight into his eyes with respect, until he signals her with a satisfied nod. She leans in his window for a hug. As she turns to go, I raise the glass. Quickly, she rushes back and smacks a kiss that leaves an imprint on the window for us to keep until she returns. I can see the sadness in Hugh's eyes as he searches the black squares of the bus to see where Mary is seated as it pulls away. For a moment, he looks desperate; he can't find her. Then the bus is gone.

We're down to three. Once home, Anna retreats upstairs with an enormous bowl of chocolate chip cookie dough ice cream, her comfort food. I hear loud music behind her locked door. In the living room, Hugh turns on the television and dozes off. The phone ringing only makes his eyes flutter momentarily. It's Michaelle, his speech therapist from HealthSouth. I had asked her to call about Hugh's recent exhaustion and confusion. "Rosemary, in light of his recent testing, I don't think you can expect him to go back to work for at least a year," she says.

"What about driving? Will he ever be able to drive again?" I ask.

"Possibly, but it will take a very long time. Hang in there. Time will tell," she says. I don't even mention the call to Hugh.

On Tuesday there is no rehab. "Let's have some fun," I say to my two bored housemates. "Mary's having fun, so why can't we?" It is too hot to be outside, but the mall is cool and comfortable. We shuffle through the food court to American Eagle where Hugh finds a stray plastic chair and plops down right outside the dressing room. Anna needs new blue jeans. She tries on several pairs with different shirts, strutting like a model in a fashion show for Hugh. At the cash register, he beams down at Anna who is whispering, "Thank you Daddy," as he hands over his debit card. This is the first time he had made a purchase himself since the accident.

On Friday, while meeting with Dr. Ward's nurse practitioner for a pre-op exam, the phone rings. After the call, she says, "That was a therapist from HealthSouth trying to reach the doctor. Apparently, Hugh's scores have gone down in the last week and they want the surgeon to be aware of the change."

"What does this mean?" I ask.

"They wonder if the operation should be postponed. Maybe there is a medical reason, possibly another brain bleed. He'll need a CAT scan."

I feel sick. Could he really have another bleed out of the blue after three months? Hugh and I are both ready for this operation to be over. The test is immediately set up for the following Monday morning with the surgical plan contingent upon Hugh showing no significant brain swelling. The nurse practitioner continues, "This may have to do with anxiety. Anxiety in TBI patients manifests itself physically, especially at the early stages of recuperation. Relax this weekend. We'll know more on Monday."

I look at her feeling dizzy. *Relax? I feel like manifesting physically right now too, like passing out, but we have another appointment.*

"I really think this is anxiety, Mrs. Rawlins," she says as if reading my mind. "Try not to worry too much. Good luck!"

With that, we head out the door to see the anesthesiologist, who administers an EKG and gives Hugh a clean bill of health to proceed with the operation. Soon we're home again, waiting, still not knowing whether or not Hugh will have his head repaired.

The weekend drags, so we try to stay busy. Kevin and his daughter visit. He assembles a homemade pulley that he's devised for Hugh to strengthen his shoulder while two-year old Caleigh plays dress-up with Anna's old dance outfits. She twirls and spins for Hugh and giggles as her silky jazz skirt swirls around her tiny legs. Kevin sets Hugh up in a chair below the pulley and shows him how to grab the handles and pull one side then the other to help his range of motion and develop muscle for swimming again.

The alarm rings at six-thirty on Monday morning. Anna joins us for the ride to MCV for Hugh's CT scan. Because we arrive early, they take us right away. A few hours later at home, the phone rings.

"Everything looks fine, Mrs. Rawlins," the doctor says. "He can have the operation."

I send up a prayer of thanks, hang up the phone and turn to Hugh. "Great news! It's all set. Are you ready for surgery?"

He looks at my face with a look so deep and lost I lean into him for a tight hug.

"Are you scared?" I ask.

"They're operating on my brain!" he says.

"It's more like the area over your brain, putting your cap back on. I think you'll feel better once it's done."

"I guess. You know I don't like the hospital," he says. "But I want to get it over with." Lee stops by in the evening and promises to back up our alarm with a phone call since the surgery is so early in the morning.

"Try to get some rest," he tells us when he leaves.

Hugh is unusually pensive all evening. "I hope you know how much I love you," he says before falling asleep.

Chapter 29

Rosemary and Hugh,

Thanks for the update. Good luck! I'm sure Hugh will miss the "divot" in some perverse way.

Brett

-CFO of Hugh's company

Three months out

Lee calls the house at exactly five a.m. as promised. We dress quickly and skip breakfast. Hugh is quiet and calm as we drive with Anna to the hospital. Once we arrive on the surgical floor, a nurse takes over. "Ready Mr. Rawlins?" she asks in a chipper voice. His face already looks sleepy, as if he's preparing to be put under.

Electra arrives by eight bearing a cup of coffee and a Ghirardelli dark candy bar for me. "Sorry if I'm feeding your addiction," she jokes. Hugh's parents meet us, and together we wait for news. By ten thirty the surgery is over. "We have successfully removed the fruit bowl from Hugh's head," Dr. Ward announces cheerfully. He tells me he expects that Hugh's headaches will subside now. The skull section that had been on ice in the hospital freezer for more than three months is reattached. Hugh can now ditch the helmet. Anna and I take turns sitting by Hugh as he wades in and out of a pharmaceutical sleep.

The following day, Hugh is nauseated and throwing up. He has not eaten, but he needs to eat and keep food down before being discharged. The drain is still in his head. Anna curls up in bed beside him.

We are hoping he'll come home today, the same day as Mary, but the anti-nausea meds are making him too groggy to eat. I do something I never thought I could ever do: I hold Hugh's head while a doctor pulls out his drain and staples. Without flinching, I watch the drain slide out like bloody spaghetti. I'm euphoric at having stayed upright. I wish my older brother, John, could see me now!

Anna and I do not want to be at the hospital. The antiseptic smell brings back vivid memories we'd rather forget. Since Anna doesn't have Mary for company, I spend time walking the city streets with her while Hugh sleeps. Just down the block we meander through the Valentine Museum's garden. On the way back, I am so glad to have her soft hand in mine, and her reassuring smile that is less and less like a child's every day.

Mary arrives home late at night bursting with stories to share. Her face is radiantly happy. It changes instantly when she hears that her dad is not home yet. "Show us your pictures!" Anna says. Mary perks up again. But while Anna and I listen to her, we yawn. As we try to keep our tired eyes open after a long day at the hospital, I can see the sadness of our house seeping back into Mary. We'll be back to the hospital tomorrow... here we go again...here comes the forced, quiet routine of recuperation.

We wake at six-thirty to go to MCV where we find Hugh able to walk the hall and eat. His eyes light up when he spots Mary standing in the doorway and she runs to him. Once home, Hugh is anxious to call Kevin. In a new firm voice, I hear him say, "Now we'll have to go head to head and do battle!"

"Those are *fighting* words," I say, when he hangs up.

"I feel whole again. It's weird, but now I feel like I can get down to business."

I squeeze his arm. "Uh oh! Watch out, everyone!" I say, laughing.

It's Anna's turn for a mini vacation. She has been invited to the beach with her friend Christie's family. Mary bakes an anniversary cake for Hugh's parents and we surprise them with a lunch celebration at their house. "Hugh seems different to me," his mother remarks.

"He is," I say. "He's more confident. Cross your fingers!" She nods enthusiastically at me. Afterward, I remind Hugh to do his wall push-ups, expecting him to be too tired. He completes ten on the wall with no help, a new record.

By Monday night, he is much clearer. We are getting ready for our evening walk after dinner. When I run downstairs, I see him sitting at the kitchen table *tying his own sneakers*! I cannot believe my eyes. It's as if he had never lost the use of his left hand. He's leaning over in the chair too, and not getting dizzy. I am breathless. "Look Hugh. Look what you're doing!"

"I'm tying my sneakers," he says, barely glancing up.

"Oh my God, I can't believe it. Can you hold a pen with your left hand?" I ask. "Can you write?"

"I don't know. I guess." Rifling through the kitchen desk drawer, I find a pen and quickly hand it to him. He writes his name with his left hand. My eyes tear up. Hugh looks mortified. "You're embarrassing me," he complains. "All I did was sign my name."

"Hugh, don't you realize, you could *not* do that before?"

"I guess," he shrugs.

I'm dumbfounded. His left side has made a miraculous comeback. Dr. Ward said it sometimes happens that way; it's not known exactly why. Perhaps it's partly emotional. Hugh says he feels like he has been "put back together again." I look forward to seeing his old determination return full force.

Hugh starts rehab again full-time, attending Monday through Friday, nine to one-thirty. Again, he is provided rides to and from rehab. Cathy, his cognitive/speech therapist, says he's a little behind but should be fine in a week or so.

Electra jumps back in to help. She's massaging Hugh. "Wow," she says, "I can't believe how much muscle tone he has lost from being immobile for just a week." Mary and Anna's friends have grown accustomed to seeing Hugh sprawled out on the family room floor as Electra digs her elbows into his back while she talks to me. Hugh is thin, somewhere in the 150s with no appetite, but he's beginning to show signs that he wants more activity.

The cycling gang has chipped in to replace Hugh's bike frame, so Kevin takes Hugh out bike shopping. He also gives Hugh some exercises to do at home to strengthen his arms and legs and improve his balance.

"Are you sure this is a good idea?" I ask them. The idea of Hugh riding a bike is alarming to me.

"Yes," says Hugh firmly. "It's a stationary bike for now," Kevin assures me.

"Are you sure you don't want to take up Parcheesi?" I ask. Eyes roll all around.

"I don't want Dad to ever ride his bike on the road again," Mary says to me at night in the kitchen.

"I feel the same way. We'll have to work through this as a family when the time comes. For now, he's using a stationary bike and I can live with that." She stares at me before looking away.

Hugh's dexterity has improved, but his stamina is still a problem. Many of Hugh's friends don't realize just how tired he is and how much rest he needs. Understandably, everyone still expects him to be the pre-injury Hugh who pushed himself to the limit. But Hugh tells me he's tired from the inside out, so dead tired he can barely stand at times. He seldom does the exercises Kevin shows him. In truth, rehab knocks him out. When I give him his "to do" list of exercises, he puts it on the table and quietly says, "Maybe later," before falling asleep.

What has grown is his desire to do more. His mother is right. I can see that even though he's tired, he's changed. It's as though he's made a decision. He says he wants to be more alert, he wishes he had the energy to exercise. Maybe this is the first step, the wanting. I know if he wants something enough, no one will work harder.

Chapter 30

Three months out

Our lawyer, Liz, now calls frequently because the woman who hit Hugh is due to appear in traffic court soon. The week before, she calls to tell me it will be beneficial to have the entire family in court so the judge can see Hugh's wife and children at his side. "It won't hurt to see that bandage on Hugh's head from the surgery either," she says. "Visuals always help."

The phone rings again as I dig through the pantry for a makeshift dinner. "You won't believe this, Rosemary, but our star witness was not subpoenaed for some reason," Liz says, exasperated.

"I believe it," I say.

"Anyway, I called him and he agreed to come to court. His name is Wray. He was the driver directly behind the woman who hit Hugh. He saw everything."

"That's really nice of him," I say relieved.

"It is. He promised me he'll be there…and, well, there's one other thing," Liz says, and pauses. "Would you be willing to describe the extent of Hugh's injuries in court, if they ask? I think it would be most effective if you did the talking, but no pressure. If it's too much…"

"I'll do it," I say. After hanging up, I wonder if I should have thought about it more. The girls will hear his prognosis. I'll have to be graphic and brutally honest.

The day before the traffic court hearing, Hugh falls into a deep sleep on the couch in my office in the afternoon and awakes disoriented. He will not talk to Mary or me. Using hand signals, he points to things or shrugs. "What's wrong with Dad today?" Mary whispers.

Rubbing his forearm, I prod him, "What is it? Is your head hurting?" I ask. Hugh's face is lined with distress. He leans forward, elbows on his knees, hands clasped.

"What if she says it was my fault?" he asks. He has no memory whatsoever about that day, or even several days before the accident. Lowering his head, he whispers, "What kind of moron gets hit by a car while riding his bike?"

"The kind that doesn't have eyes in back of his head," I answer. "Hugh, you were in the right place. You did nothing wrong. Everyone said so. You've been riding safely every week for almost twenty years. Doesn't that tell you something?"

He turns his head toward me, eyes fired up, "How could she not see me there? I had on my cycling jersey!" I'm glad to see him angry instead of despondent.

"I don't know. All I know is that you were always careful. She wasn't paying attention. She was charged with reckless driving, endangering another. The police said it was *her* fault."

It grates on Hugh that he cannot remember what happened. Now I see how hard he's been trying to remember, to reconstruct the day, the series of events that robbed him of so much.

"I did this to you and the girls," he says, a single tear streaking his face.

"This is not your fault! All you've ever done is love us and take care of us," I say. "If you want to stay home, you can…"

"I'll go," he whispers, smothering me in a hug.

Before court, Hugh has a post-surgical appointment to be readmitted to rehab at HealthSouth. As he walks down the PT corridor, Jennifer runs out of her office to hug him. Penny, Michaelle, and Cathy follow a minute later. Soon, a small crowd gathers together watching as Hugh extends his left hand to Penny. As she shakes his hand, her face lights up at his tighter grasp. She meets his eyes with an admiring stare, and says, "Looks like you've got it back. We'll be working on that!" Hugh smiles broadly. A quick meeting with Dr. G. sets him up to continue in all therapies.

After this upbeat reunion, I drive Hugh back home to pick up the girls and his parents for the trip to General District Court where we are on the morning docket. We file in one by one, empty our pockets, and pose with arms extended as security officers wave their wands over us. Once through the security archway, Liz guides us to the courtroom where we are seated in the third row with her husband, Ken, and Keith, our minister, who has joined us for moral support.

Finally, we see the woman who hit Hugh, the woman who has caused so many mixed emotions in me. At first, I pitied her. Poor little old lady, I thought, she must be completely shaken up and haunted by this accident. Then, when we never heard a word from her, I questioned her conscience. Friends told me that lawyers always counsel their clients not to speak to the victim, but I can't get over the fact that there has not been one attempt to convey any concern to us.

There she stands in profile, the woman who made a split second mistake that changed the entire future of my family. Dressed conservatively, standing submissively, I can't explain why she reminds me of Carol Channing. Her face is hard to read. She does not appear nervous or regretful. I can't gauge her expression, so I stare at her, wishing I could turn away. Then it comes to me. She looks bored—bored and a little annoyed. Her lawyer speaks in a sympathetic voice. He tells the judge that this was just a terrible mistake, a tragic accident.

The judge's voice springs me to attention. He's questioning the only eyewitness, Wray. Looking uncomfortable, Wray shifts his weight nervously. His voice shakes as he describes the positions of the cars and Hugh. He testifies that Hugh was hit directly from behind. Halfway through his testimony, he chokes up. "I'm sorry," he says, swallowing a sob. "I will never forget these images for as long as I live." A lawyer asks him to name *exactly* where the car was in relation to the bike. It feels to me like the lawyer is trying to make him contradict himself.

He tells the court that when the car hit Hugh, he went over the hood and flew 150 feet in the air before hitting the road. He says the woman just sat in the car while he called 911. She asked him, "What did I hit?" as if not knowing she hit a person. He says he could not look at Hugh. He was afraid to see what Hugh looked like, but he heard him screaming, and said he has had nightmares about it ever since.

I sit in the third row with Hugh, his parents, and our girls listening, imagining, trying not to pass out; worried that I'll be called next and I might not be able to speak.

The officer's testimony comes next. Her statements corroborate with the witness. She confirms that the driver said she had no idea what she hit. She tells the court where the car was, where Hugh landed on the road.

On follow-up, the driver's lawyer does not have anything to say except that this was a tragic accident. I lean forward, trying to remember what I might say if asked, trying to string together some sentences in my head, when the judge voices his verdict.

I never get to say a word.

"Guilty of improper driving," the judge announces. A small fine is charged. Done.

What? I walk over to our lawyer. Reading devastation on my face, she puts her arm around me. "This is good news, Rosemary," she says. "She's been found guilty and this will be good for our case—for the insurance."

"But what about the reckless charge?" Suddenly, I want that word in there. It seems insane that she's not charged with anything more. *Improper* driving? What does that mean? *Improper* is when you put your elbows on the table during a meal, not when you run someone over with your car because you weren't paying attention! Liz assures me it's a good verdict. She steers me away from the bench and toward the family. We all quietly exit the courtroom. Outside in the hall, we meet Wray, the witness who spoke on Hugh's behalf. As he shakes Hugh's hand, he openly cries, "I'm so sorry. I wish I could have helped more. I wanted to help more." Hugh is speechless, but nods at the man. "You have a beautiful family," Wray says to Hugh.

"We are so grateful you came," I say. "Thank you for stopping that day. Thank you for coming today." He looks at Hugh, at the girls, and tears build in his eyes again. "You didn't have to come, but you came anyway. It means a lot." I try to reassure him. He hugs me in the hall.

"I'll never forget this. If I can ever do anything for you, please call me," he says. We break apart to the sound of laughter. It's the woman who hit Hugh walking away with her lawyer. She's laughing out loud, no doubt because she got off easy. Our whole group sees her. Our jaws fall open in disbelief.

All the compassion I felt for this woman before I ever saw her disappears and is replaced by a sickening ball of hatred in the pit of my stomach. I now feel like an idiot for preaching to my children about not judging people prematurely.

Liz walks up beside me and says, "It's over. At least they weren't granted a continuance. I'll deal with the insurance company and keep you informed." She hugs all of us warmly before leaving.

The day before the court date, I had gotten an allergy shot; I was a few weeks late for it. As I climb into the Explorer after leaving the courthouse, my arm itches uncontrollably. While scratching it, I notice my entire upper left arm turning an angry red. I drive everyone home and set out an impromptu lunch. At the table, I can feel my upper arm swelling. Once Hugh's parents say their good-byes and head home, I rub some cortisone on my arm to calm the itch, but a short while later a tennis ball sized lump bulges above my elbow. Since I am asthmatic, a serious reaction is possible. Mary insists I go to the doctor immediately and quickly puts on her shoes to come with me. It's the last thing I want to do right now.

Hugh is sprawled in the recliner, drained from his hectic day. A quick tilt of Anna's head and her eyes tell me she will stay close to Hugh while I'm gone. In the car, Mary talks down my anxiety. I'm actually more worried about being out of commission for the family than I am about my own health. It turns out that the swelling is just a local reaction and goes away in a few days with Benadryl. I still wonder if my pent up anger from the courtroom built up in my body when I couldn't yell at the judge. I imagine over and over again saying to him, "I'd like to see a woman run over *your* wife and almost kill her, and see how you feel about the phrase *improper driving*!"

Later, Keith calls. "Just checking up on you," he says with concern. "It was more painful seeing you in that courtroom than in the ICU."

"Keith, I know I'm angry because of what she did. But did you see any compassion or sorrow in that woman's face today? Maybe I just couldn't see it. You're a minister, I'm sure you noticed something."

"I'm sorry, Rosemary, I didn't. I have to say, it's really shocking. It was sad. The witness was much more shaken up then she was."

I hang up the phone, my teeth clenched, heart racing. I know I have no room for this anger in my heart. I have enough to deal with and need to stay healthy. I have long equated pent up anger and hatred with cancer, like a debilitating disease that cripples and maims. I will not let this woman make me ill. I pray for the strength to let my anger go.

Hugh's Uncle Link told us, "Look to the stars." I still do, but I wonder sometimes if they are pulling away from us. Hugh and I have been humbled. Life is unpredictable, not the controllable sequence of events we thought we had all figured out. People aren't what they seem. My once pristine view of the world and the people in it has been shaken.

"I worried about her," I later say to Hugh. "I honestly worried about that awful woman. How can you seem so calm about her?"

"Because shit happens," he says. "Remember when I said that to Keith when he asked me what I thought about the accident?"

"Yes, you're always so poetic," I say, rolling my eyes.

"It's how I choose to look at it. Sometimes all the analyzing in the world won't make our bad feelings go away. All we can do is move on. I'm moving on—how about you?"

"I'll try." The words stick in my throat.

Chapter 31

Four months out

Hugh worked as Assistant Controller for a Fortune 500 company in Richmond before he was hurt. He had over sixty people reporting to him.

As soon as his boss, Tom, heard about the accident, he rushed to the hospital. I was not in the ICU at the time, but he saw Hugh and talked to Krista. Because of the severity of Hugh's injury, and under the advice of doctors, I limited visitors. I didn't personally know Tom very well. I had only met him at a couple of company parties. When I spoke to him on the phone, he was devastated.

Soon after Hugh's accident, I met Tom at lunch in the bustling cafeteria at MCV. As we sat at a small table speckled with crumbs, he presented me with a beautiful basket of food and information about

Hugh's benefits and pay structure during his hospital stay. He expected to hear a full report.

"Tom, the doctors can't give me definitive answers about Hugh's recovery. There's not much I can tell you right now, except that it may take time," I told him. "But I'm worried. I worked in the HR field years ago. I know these things take on a life of their own. At first, everyone is shocked and offers help; they continue this way for a while until work piles up and people get restless. But eventually they give up on the employee. I'm told that this is going to be a very long road, a slow recovery—"

Tom interrupted, "Rosemary, I want Hugh back. Don't worry. I'll do my best to hang in there for you. Hugh is an extremely valuable employee. I'll take care of him." His words put my mind at ease for the moment.

Dealing with Hugh's work associates was complicated in the early days of his injury, since I didn't know many of them well. Hugh was a professional who kept his personal and work life separate. I was now the "spokesperson" for my husband and the link to his employer. Should I tell them the doctors did not want to make any promises, that Hugh might never return to work? I had already read that many people with injuries like Hugh's wind up bagging groceries or performing simple repetitive tasks for income.

Hugh's administrative assistant, Michelle, made frequent trips to the house and worked hard to make sure I had paychecks, insurance information, and phone numbers. Many of Hugh's managers and employees wanted to visit him. I decided to draft a letter.

May 4th, 2002
Dear Friends and Colleagues of Hugh's,
As many of you know, on April 13th, Hugh suffered devastating multiple injuries after being struck by a car on his bicycle. Since that day, he and his family—and I know many of you—have been on a journey of sorts to pull him back to us. I want you to know that your thoughts, prayers, cards, gifts, and notes have been a constant reminder to us of how very precious our connection is to one another in times of need.

Hugh is well on the path to recovery. His injuries are unlike typical injuries in that no real date can be set as to when he will be able to return to work or resume the life he left on April 13. I only know he has been ahead of the curve every step of the way, shocking and surprising doctors, nurses and us with his strength, determination, and ability to constantly beat the odds. For the time being, visitors are limited to family, but I will be sure to let you know when that is changed. This is due to "doctor's orders" that greatly benefit his recuperation. When visitation resumes, I expect it will be in small groups of one or two at a time for a while. I will let you know about that also and will be happy to arrange for visits with those of you who wish to see him. Please keep in mind that progress is measured in weeks and months rather than minutes and be patient with us.

Thank you all for your incredible support. It's very heartwarming to see a corporation with a heart, a company that truly knows how to care for its employees like family. Special thanks to Tom, Brett, and Michelle. I have lost a lot of weight, Brett, and your brownies are restoring my strength! Tom and Michelle, you have been there every step of the way. I'm sorry I don't know each and every one of you who sent my husband a card, plant, basket, or prayer but I'm sure he knows all of you, and has felt your support within – I'm certain it's part of the strength he draws upon daily.

With our thanks and love,
Rosemary, Anna and Mary

Tom sent cards and gifts and stayed in touch by email and phone. One night at suppertime, he stopped by with a dozen baseball hats from Hugh's friends at work. I tried my best to keep him informed but, in truth, I avoided him. I was terrified of his reaction to all of Hugh's deficits and what that would mean for Hugh's professional future and our family's welfare. I was determined to protect Hugh and his job. By May 30th, I could no longer put Tom off. He was coming for a visit at the house.

"Hugh, this is an important visit. Try to stay focused on what Tom says, okay?" I said. Hugh was watching a sitcom and tuned me out. Earlier in the day I helped him dress in khakis and a button-down shirt. "You are so skinny, this shirt balloons all over you," I commented. "Here, try this," we switched to a golf shirt. For all my fussing, Hugh seemed unconcerned about his boss visiting.

At last minute, I decided not to use the gait belt or helmet. In my effort to make things appear better than they were, I coached Hugh to stay seated so he wouldn't fall, and urged him to focus on what Tom said.

Right on time, Tom arrived. He stepped in the foyer and strode over to Hugh's chair, putting out his hand. "I would have come sooner but your wife wouldn't let me," he said in a jovial voice. I laughed uncomfortably and showed him to the couch.

The awkward scene unfolded like a badly produced play. I don't know what Tom was thinking, but I imagined he was taken aback by Hugh's condition. At that time, Hugh was still struggling with words. He was straining to keep up with conversation and faking his way through a lot of it. Tom tried to talk business as usual. I didn't allow them any time alone and I had the feeling that bothered Tom. I stayed in the room out of fear. Fear that Tom would see Hugh's situation as hopeless. Fear that Hugh would slip and fall while trying to get out of his chair. Above all, I was afraid of Tom's report about Hugh's condition to higher management the next day.

Hugh acted remote. At times he responded to Tom's gregarious stories with a short laugh, but sometimes he stared into space. While Tom sat on the couch and talked to Hugh, my mind drifted to the updated evaluation I had received that day at HealthSouth: Hugh's attention span was ten minutes long.

Tom's voice jarred me back, as he told Hugh, "Don't get too comfortable in that chair, buddy. There's a lot of work waiting for you when you feel better!" He rose, shook Hugh's hand and I walked him to the door. "Be sure and keep me informed, Rosemary," he said. "Anything you need, just give me a call."

"Sure, Tom. Thanks for coming," I said. I could not read his face. He seemed earnest enough, truly concerned about Hugh. But work is work, I thought.

Hugh's vacation time had been used up; we were entering the short-term disability phase. There were forms to fill out and deliver to HealthSouth. After Dr. G signed them, I personally drove them to Hugh's HR Department. I met with two managers in HR to review Hugh's benefit package and paycheck policy. I signed form after form. Everyone at Hugh's workplace expressed words of encouragement and support. They said they all wanted Hugh back. Everyone I had spoken to at the hospital and at rehab cautioned against setting our hearts on his old job. I wanted to remain positive and believe he'd be a rare success story. On the other hand, I wanted to be realistic and not make him feel he had to live up to some super-hero image.

Co-workers began visiting Hugh at our house. One manager who reported to Hugh, came over one evening with 8 x 10 photos of all Hugh's coworkers holding up "I Miss You" signs. Seated in chairs or posing in the parking lot, employees beamed into the camera, each holding their personal message to Hugh. Hugh was visibly moved by this demonstration of affection. It touched him deeply. There was one picture of Tom with "I miss you" posters taped all over his body. I knew he felt Hugh's absence acutely at the office. Hugh was his trusted deputy.

I began to wonder about this other life Hugh had—his personal office life. Years ago, I had worked in an office. I remembered the alliances and camaraderie, the spats and feuds that arise from the claustrophobia of close quarters and stifling cubicles, the unavoidable power plays between colleagues, and the pride in being counted on to beat a deadline or achieve a promotion. Hugh entered that world every day and had so many relationships in which I played no part.

Co-worker visits at our home were uncomfortable for me. I was making idle conversation in our living room with people I didn't know. If Hugh was tired after rehab he barely spoke, or he'd turn on cartoons and let them blare as his colleagues squirmed uneasily nearby. It was unsettling—a grown man laughing at juvenile antics—especially someone who once read the *Wall Street Journal* cover to cover every day. Some visitors looked pensive and understanding, others looked profoundly sad. Some became dear friends. Others drifted away without as much as another phone call.

One afternoon, Tom came to our house for lunch with another manager from the office. I ordered a takeout pizza for lunch because I didn't want these men to see that Hugh could not hold an eating utensil in his left hand without extreme difficulty. He could manage a slice of pizza with two hands using mostly his right hand. The three men sat around the kitchen table. Hugh had a lot of difficulty eating. He was in his pocketing phase, storing food in his cheek, and forgetting to swallow.

After serving drinks, I left the room, but listened in from my office down the hall. All of a sudden I heard Hugh coughing. I peeked out and saw that he had spewed pizza on Tom, who was now vigorously wiping his shirt. As he cleaned up, Tom tried to make light of the situation by joking, "Gee, Hugh, you didn't have to go and spit your lunch out on me, did you?" I looked over. Hugh was smiling that awful smile of embarrassment and wiping his face with a napkin.

After everyone left and I was cleaning up, I asked Hugh how he thought it went.

"Weird," he said.

"In what way?"

"I felt self-conscious. They talked too fast. It didn't feel like old times," he said.

"Did you feel like the odd man out? Does it make you miss work?" I asked.

"Not really. They mean well, but I felt like an idiot when I coughed all over Tom. Things just feel different now. I don't know." I could sense he was disturbed by the entire meeting and felt disappointed, but wasn't sure why.

The big picture was emerging in Hugh's mind, the clash between his old reality and his new circumstances. When he was at home or at therapy he felt natural with his injury, but the contrast was stark when he was among his business peers. At rehab and at home, we had developed an understanding of Hugh's needs and adapted to his pace, but others did not know what we knew, so they couldn't make allowances.

On July 18, 2002, I received an email from Tom that read:

Thanks for the update. All our thoughts and prayers are with Hugh, you, Mary and Anna! A day does not go by when I do not think about Hugh whether at work or home. It was great talking with Hugh the other day. We truly miss him and need him. No question about that.

Some food for thought:

I have been thinking about a "return plan" for Hugh for some time. I am not trying to rush Hugh back to the office before he is ready but I believe this will work. When Hugh is ready to come back, in two or three months it would not have to start at 8 hours a day or even 5 days a week. We can play this by ear and start slow. The upside to this is:

-I will lighten his workload accordingly.

- I believe we at the office can be an important part of Hugh's recovery process.

-Hugh may not be 100% of the pre April 13th Hugh; whatever % Hugh's physical and mental capacity is when he returns I am confident he will add value to the team.

-I drive by your house every day so I would be happy to bring Hugh in every morning. We can also make arrangements to bring him home early each day. There are many people who would love to help every day.

-bottom line is a "win" for everybody.

Give it some thought and when you have a spare moment, I would be happy to meet you for coffee, breakfast or lunch and discuss further. Take care! Tom

I had no idea how to handle this. Hugh was clearly not ready for work yet. On the other hand, this was so uplifting. For now, I just let it be and thanked him.

After Hugh's skull repair, on the day he had forty staples removed from his head, I received a package on the front porch. It was a gift certificate to a Day Spa for me with a card signed by all of Hugh's A/P and accounting employees. My hand shook as I read the card with so many signatures. All these employees had been waiting a long time for news, and Tom deserved an honest explanation.

It's been nearly four months since Hugh last reported to work. I decide to call Tom and lay down the hard truth over lunch. On the second of August, we meet at Rockola Café. I ask Hugh to come, but he says he'll stay home. He's still having problems with pocketing and hates eating out.

Tom greets me warmly. After ordering drinks, I talk to him frankly. "Tom, I need to be totally honest with you. Hugh is still struggling with this injury; it affects a lot of what he does at work."

"Whatever it is, Rosemary, we can work with it. We just want him back."

"Look at this," I say as I slide a piece of paper across the lunch table. It's a list of Hugh's deficits—a long list. As Tom scans the note, his expression contorts; he rubs both sides of his face, leans against the leather-backed booth, and bursts into tears. "I'm so sorry," he cries. "This is just so hard to hear. It's so sad."

I am walking a tightrope. I wonder how much I should expose. No one knows what to expect in terms of recovery; there's no prognosis or timeline. I can tell that Tom misses Hugh at the office, but it's the *healthy* Hugh he misses. I know he is trying hard to do the right thing, but work is piling up, he has deadlines, and has to make decisions. On the other hand, he has made a promise to me. He said he wouldn't give up on Hugh. I'm also aware that this is a promise he may not be in control of keeping.

I decide to talk to Lee Facetti about this. Lee was Hugh's boss a few years back and knows Hugh professionally as well as personally. I know he'll be able to offer me an objective view of where Hugh's capabilities really lie at this point. Lee decides to see what Hugh can do. Over the weekend, he and Hugh review their real estate business. Hugh has trouble checking over spreadsheets and using the computer. His dexterity is not fine-tuned yet, so using the mouse is slow, and he becomes confused trying to sift through all the information on the computer screen. Lee is respectful; he allows Hugh time and never comments on the difficulties he encounters. While Hugh is fairly articulate, he still can't concentrate beyond short periods.

"Rosemary," Lee says, "I'm sure that Hugh's knowledge is still there. It's just his processing that's slow. I really think with therapy and time, he'll improve."

Hugh's brain is slowly rewiring itself to go from dial up service to high speed Internet. It doesn't happen overnight.

Chapter 32

Dear Liz,

I have done a total 360 regarding that woman. She was laughing as she left the courthouse and looking very smug, and believe me, I am a person who gives EVERYBODY the benefit of the doubt. What happens now?

Rosemary

-Email to my lawyer

Five months out

The insurance company does not want to pay us the maximum amount of damages. I receive discovery papers in the mail from the lawyer representing the woman who hit Hugh, a stack of twenty-five pages of detailed questions. I must document every doctor visit Hugh has had for the past ten years, provide his entire employment history, and request his tax returns. Digging through old records in the attic feels like annoying busy work when I have so many other things to do. We have yet to hear one word from the opposing company. They haven't even offered to reimburse us for Hugh's demolished bike.

I think about the house we bought only eighteen months before his accident, the biggest house we've ever owned. I wanted it so much. Now it's just a financial burden with more space to clean.

Hugh has also asked about driving. A phone call from the Health-South case manager informs us that driver re-training won't be recommended for "a good six months." Hugh slides into a funk as if not driving is the most serious of our worries. "I know I can drive. Just give me a chance," he says.

"It's not up to me," I tell him, with an edge in my voice, as I pick up the phone to talk to a lady in his HR department from work. She has good news: Hugh is entitled to a full sixty percent of his old salary for up to two years through the disability plan. We are also told they owe us a few vacation checks. I shoot Hugh a high five when I hang up. "Never thought we'd be so happy about a pay cut," he laughs.

On August 25th, I'm told at rehab that I should prepare Hugh for the possibility that he may never return to his old job. There is talk of a plateau. Hugh's left side is slowly improving, but his speed and initiation are still big problems. This plateau is not necessarily permanent, but the therapists feel that preparing emotionally for job loss is important, just in case.

Nancy Foley tells me about a Rehabilitation Community in Virginia. This residential program would help Hugh regain independent living skills and receive vocational rehab. He would be expected to dress, cook, eat, clean, and attend therapy sessions in a supervised environment until he was able to take care of himself. The only drawback I see is that he would live away from us. The facility is over an hour away. With the girls in school, we wouldn't be able to visit much.

"I don't think Hugh would get out of bed if we weren't around," I say. "What if he didn't remember and thought we had abandoned him?"

"The staff is caring there, and they would surely remind him he was not alone," Nancy says. "It's just an option and many people benefit greatly from it. Just keep it in the back of your mind if Hugh continues to linger on this plateau."

This conversation worries me deeply. I keep Hugh on his therapy schedule at HealthSouth while stepping things up at home by making more demands on him. I read with him and ask him to look things up for me. I enlist the girls' help too.

As Mary sits at the kitchen table with Hugh, she holds a workbook open in front of him. It shows three pictures: a dog, a cat, and a car. "Which one doesn't match, Dad?"

"The cat?"

Mary swings her head to me, eyes wide, and tries again. Anna asks

Hugh for help with her math homework. We all force him to focus several times a day.

Ten days later the story changes completely. All reports are positive. Hugh is progressing again, so he's put back into full-time therapy. Even though he's running out of paid visits, I sign him up and decide we'll find a way to pay for it later. Dr. G also suggests he try a new drug called Amantadine that has helped other patients increase their focus and attention.

The Long Term Disability people tell us to file for disability benefits "the sooner, the better." I am informed it is a lengthy process involving a determination period, and almost no one is accepted on the first try. Another mound of paperwork ensues. At the same time, I begin writing my own résumé in case I need a job with benefits soon.

I'm sitting in Nancy Foley's office when she informs me that the cost of Hugh's combined therapies will run $600 a day once the HMO no longer agrees to pay. The figure is so staggering, I laugh out loud. My heart races all afternoon thinking about what that will add up to in a month if he goes five days a week. I look out the window of Applebee's during lunch with a friend and see a homeless person walking down Broad Street pushing his possessions in a decrepit grocery cart. "That could be me in a year," I mutter.

I remember something my husband taught me: everything is negotiable. I call the bookkeeping department and meet with an accountant at HealthSouth to discuss cost-cutting strategies. I ask the therapists to cut down to three times a week as soon as they can, but not so much that it will compromise Hugh's progress. I wonder how people with little or no insurance ever make it through an injury like this. I later discover that, on average, TBI patients receive about one to two months of therapy before being left on their own. Hugh is one of the fortunate few to receive ongoing care.

Our application is forwarded to the Disability Determination Board. It's accepted on the first try—another reminder that Hugh's condition is dire. I don't know if I should be happy or sad about the news.

On September 13th, I roll over in bed and wake Hugh up with a kiss. "Happy Birthday, Hon. You almost didn't make this one." In the evening, our doorbell rings. Michelle and Dixie are standing on the stoop holding a huge birthday basket adorned with helium balloons and stuffed with gifts from twenty-five people at the office. Hugh laughs with them in the hallway. "Thanks! Tell everyone I miss them," he says.

When Michelle and Dixie leave, I help Hugh hurry to get ready. His cycling friends are throwing a surprise party for him too—a boy's night out. He thinks he's only having dinner with Rick. While they're gone, Lara stays with me. We sit on my candlelit front porch with a bottle of wine and talk as the September sky turns from blue to streaks of yellow, orange and black. "Where are the girls?" Lara asks.

"They had plans with friends tonight," I say. "We'll have a family dinner with Hugh's parents tomorrow. Hugh gets to have a two-day birthday this year. I think he's earned it!"

"How was your night out?" I ask Hugh when he arrives home.

"Okay," he says with little emotion. "I enjoyed it, but I'm not like them anymore."

"What do you mean?"

"They tried to include me, but they talked about their ride last weekend and their jobs. I have nothing to talk about." As I reach out to touch his arm, he turns away and walks upstairs.

A new bike is set up on a wind trainer in the garage where Hugh uses it once or twice, but doesn't like the saddle, or so he says. Holding himself up on the bike is a form of strength training, and his left arm and hand are still weak. Still, he misses the camaraderie of riding with his friends. Cycling alone in a dusty garage, hearing the wheels spin in the silence of the empty space, exaggerates his isolation. For the first time ever, he is not motivated to exercise. As much as his friends and colleagues want to include him, he is on his own. He tries some positive self-talk: "If it's to be, it's up to me," he says, as though trying to summon strength from inside.

The time has come for Hugh to give his deposition for the court case. As we drive to our lawyer's office in Richmond, Hugh does not appear nervous in the least. I am instructed to wait in the lobby while Hugh, the driver who hit him, and her passenger all deliver their statements to four different lawyers. A court reporter records their words.

As a possible witness in the case, I am not permitted to sit in on their depositions.

As each woman records her statement, the other one waits in the lobby. For twenty minutes I sit across from the woman who hit Hugh as she waits for her turn to be deposed. I notice she looks older today than she did in court. I remember her hair looking more blonde, but now it appears gray. The two of us sit silent in our own spaces, in this small room of chairs, coffee tables, and plants. In my mind, I'm convinced she knows who I am, yet she appears nonchalant. When she looks up from her magazine, I challenge her with my eyes to say something. I want her to say, "I'm so sorry, if only I could undo that one moment, I would."

That's all I want.

She says nothing—at least not to me. Her calmness makes me twitch with frustration. Finally, I conclude that her true thoughts must be *why did this boy have to run into my car and ruin my life?* After giving her deposition, the lady's passenger joins her. The two women sit and chat about their jewelry and the weather. I want to scream in their faces. "Screw your jewelry! Screw you!"

Oblivious to me, their lawyer walks in and out of the lobby. He pats the driver's hand sympathetically and whispers words of comfort in her ear.

A rage builds in me. I picture myself in her face yelling, "Look what you have done to us! Look at our life now! Are you at all concerned about the damage you've caused? Can't you see you ran over my husband? You ran over my life?"

But I squash it down.

After a while they leave. Hugh is still in the office. I remain on the love seat in the lobby reflecting on what I said earlier in the morning, "Now Hugh, please don't joke around in there. Please remember this is serious. Tell the truth about how hard it's been for you."

Liz agreed. "This is not the time to suck it up," she coached. "Tell the truth. I know the way you guys are, never admitting the pain. This is the time to tell it like it is." He gave us his goofy slanted smile and said, "I'll try."

Another ninety minutes later, the court reporter wheels out her computer equipment just ahead of Hugh. She smiles at him gaily and says, "Goodbye Mr. Rawlins. I love your sense of humor." I cut my eyes at him. He just smiles and raises his eyebrows.

"What's so funny?" I ask.

"When Hugh was asked what he studied in college, he answered, 'Girls and surfing,'" Liz says.

Feeling drained and tight enough to crack, I make a feeble effort to laugh at the joke. Liz and Hugh fill me in on the other details in her office. Basically, the women said they saw only a flash of color before hitting him. The passenger said she thought he was an orange construction cone. *Sure, a six-foot, 198-pound orange construction cone...with wheels!*

We now continue to prepare for the possible court case in the event we receive no offer of a settlement, but we hope to avoid the stress involved in a court action. Whatever we receive in the end may or may not cover the legal and medical bills that are racking up, but any amount would help. Deep inside, though, it's not her money I want, it's her remorse. I don't think any court in the land can award me that.

I drive Hugh home feeling drained, but relieved that this step in the process is over. I try again to let go of my anger toward the woman who hit him. It's clearly hurting me more than it hurts her.

"How do you feel about that woman now?" I ask.

"Indifferent. I don't even think about her. She's basically an old woman who made a terrible mistake. But she needs to pay for her mistakes," he says, with a hint of malice.

Spoken like a true accountant.

Chapter 33

Hugh,
I sure do miss getting diet cokes for you! I miss having you around.
Michelle

-Hugh's Administrative Assistant

Hugh had been in charge of accounts payable, financial reporting, and general accounting before his accident. On September 18th, I wake up to an email from Tom saying he is swamped at work and might have to hire an accounts payable director to handle Hugh's workload since five months have now gone by. We make a date for Tom to visit our home the following evening after work so he can talk to Hugh in person.

"There goes my job," Hugh says. "Next, they'll hire the rest out."

"Maybe they'll hire someone temporary," I offer, before my voice peters out.

Later in the evening we are sitting around the dinner table when we hear a knock at the front door. I peek out and it's Tom.

"Hi," I say. "I thought you were coming tomorrow night."

"I really need to talk to Hugh. I'm sorry. I can't wait any longer," he says.

I invite him in and apologize that we are eating. "Would you like to join us for dinner?"

"No thanks, but I'll take a drink if you have one." I grab him a beer and pull a desk chair up to the table. Anna and Mary continue eating quietly. Tom explains that he's stretched to the limit at work and there have been some management changes. He talks to Hugh about people they know and processes only they understand.

"Can we be excused?" Mary asks. When I nod, the girls slowly walk upstairs with a few backward glances.

Tom continues, "There is now a new president and there will be a new interim Chief Financial Officer shortly. We are really struggling to get things done without you. I need to make some changes soon."

Hugh hangs on every word and suddenly interjects, "Well, maybe I can come back and help." I shift in my chair and set down my fork.

"Could you do that, buddy?" Tom is clearly excited to hear these words.

Hugh smiles and answers, "Sure, I feel like I can help."

"That would be great! With everyone missing you so much, morale will pick up the minute you walk in the door. Every day will be good therapy for you."

"Hugh still can't drive," I interject. "What about getting to work, Tom?"

"I can pick Hugh up on my way in. It's right on my way," he states, as if that's that.

I sit dumbfounded and speechless for a minute. Then I clear my throat and say, "Is anyone remembering that Hugh is on disability? We need to check with the doctor." I realize I sound like a mother and not a wife. Tom and Hugh both look at me, then at each other with raised eyebrows. I continue anyway. "We need to take this one step at a time. Hugh can't work full time right now."

"He won't have to. He can work two to three days a week, half days to start," Tom says.

"But Tom, how long can you realistically put up with that, as busy as you are?"

"At least eight weeks," he says. "Then we can take it from there. You are being overprotective, Rosemary. Hugh will be fine. Work will be the perfect environment for him." I struggle to control my face, trying not to look so ambushed.

Hugh sits beaming at the other end of the table, happier than I've seen him in months. Tom looks at me earnestly and says, "Really, it will be great!"

I feel an avalanche coming, a foreboding. "How about I check with

HealthSouth and we'll get back to you. Okay, Tom?" I say.

After Tom leaves, I remember Dr. G saying, "Work is out of the question right now." It is estimated that Hugh should not work for a year, and even then, they will have to re-evaluate. Tom's idea is nuts, but at the same time, it's so wonderfully hopeful. Hugh's mood begins to rub off on me. Suddenly I'm grateful to Tom—maybe this is the push I need to let go. Hugh will have to try eventually, so why not now?

In bed, my mind will not stop racing to sleep. Yes, Tom's right. No, Tom's wrong. I give in and take a sleeping pill and slide down into a dark dream: we have to sell our beautiful house for a different one, but once I get inside, the new house feels all wrong and I don't like it. The floors are not level and the walls are all slanted. The carpets are matted and things look lopsided and dirty. I decide to go out in the backyard, but with each step I take, the lush green lawn turns into a sickly yellow toxic waste. I am sinking and screaming, "Get me out!" I look over toward the driveway at three well-dressed women standing there in conversation, ignoring me. I call to them, "I'm sinking in toxic waste!" They glance my way and casually resume talking. One woman swings her ponytail from side to side laughing. I slowly trudge out onto the driveway dripping with thick yellow blobs all over me. I have goop in my nails, my hair, and splattered on my shirt, but the women treat me like nothing is wrong. I am in extreme distress and nobody notices. I wake up to the loud thumping of my own heart.

Long intense discussions ensue with HealthSouth while emails flash back and forth from Hugh's company. Our disability case manager assures us that there is a graduated back-to-work program to protect us in the event the job doesn't work out. Hugh is entitled to six months of gradually working up to his old position; he will continue to collect his disability paychecks in addition to hourly wages from work up to a certain maximum amount. If it doesn't go well, he goes back on disability. It all seems too good to be true.

Hugh's personality is a huge factor in all this. He desperately wants to go back and says he is willing to accept the consequences if he cannot do the work. Telling him he cannot try is more devastating to him than letting him try and fail. Hugh is my polar opposite. I am a planner and organizer—I don't like to attempt goals that I may not achieve—and I don't like surprises. My life lately has been one big surprise, so my character has been stretched to new limits. Hugh is a risk-taker. He believes in the suitable idiom, "falling off the bike and getting right back on." Our caseworker calls him a contender. It is the perfect word for him. He has to try, even if the odds are against him. In fact, he seems to thrive on having the odds against him. If he never tries, he'll never know.

Dr. G is not convinced this will work. He strongly urges Hugh to reconsider. On the other hand, Hugh's speech therapists feel he may be up to the challenge, and with the proper conditions—cooperative staff, short hours, a familiar job, less responsibility— it could work. In addition, I assure them that the two managers who would work directly with Hugh are both top notch and his administrative assistant is the best. Dr. G reluctantly agrees under the condition that Hugh has a job coach.

Hugh and I also meet together with Nancy Foley. She tends toward Dr. G's feeling that a return to work is premature, but understands that Hugh needs to try. She reminds us that *we* are important, the couple that is Rosemary and Hugh, and urges us to follow our instincts and work together in our decision-making. We take her advice and listen intently to one another before coming to an agreement. Hugh is set on trying. I will not be the one to hold him back.

Once the decision is final, we rummage through his closet for dress clothes that might still fit. Before the accident, he wore a 38-inch waist; he's now a 32. We find some suit pants from years ago that fit. With a belt and dress shirt, they don't look half bad, so off they go to the dry cleaners.

There is a chaotic week of meetings before Hugh actually starts his job. The first time he returns to his office building is to attend a short meeting with Tom to solidify his return-to-work program. As I drive Hugh in the Explorer, he sits in the passenger seat, his olive dress pants and button-down shirt neatly pressed. Feeling jumpy inside, I ask him, "Are you nervous at all?"

"I'm more excited than nervous," he says, but he looks proud, almost jovial, an expression I have not seen on his face in months.

As we pull into the company parking lot, two of his co-workers are walking across the lawn on their way back from lunch. They see our car and glance over, hands shading their eyes to be sure they believe what they see. "Hey, you're late!" Hugh yells out the car window with his hands cupping his mouth. They wave back smiling, happy to see him. As I round the curb that lines the entrance to the large two-story building, Hugh leans over and kisses me goodbye. He steps out of the car and turns to look back at me through the window. Our eyes meet, full of promise. As I watch him enter the building with his briefcase firmly in hand, I wave. He disappears into the dark lobby, swallowed whole by the world of work—where he'll once again compete and be judged, not against who he is now, but who he was five short months ago.

I can barely choke back the odd mixture of pride and dread lodged in my throat to pull away and drive back home, alone.

Chapter 34

Back in the hospital waiting room again while you take the neuropsych evaluation. I hope this test gives you the answers you want. Go baby go!

-Notes from my journal

Six months out

Hugh arrives home with a wide grin on his face that makes me curious, because he's usually in a sour mood after his Interactive Metronome® therapy, a new therapy that has been found to improve motor planning, sequencing, and attention. Hugh has barely tolerated these sessions because they are so frustrating to him. He has to clap or tap his foot in synchronization to a metronome while a computer times his reaction. Because he dislikes the therapy so much, he does not like the therapist either. "Okay, so what's the secret?" I ask, smiling back at him.

"I was done with that stupid metronome and my brain was fried," he says. "But the therapist suggested we play basketball as a way for me to work on my left arm. I told him I wasn't in the mood, but he kept insisting and calling to me, even though I wasn't very far away. The guy yells like I'm deaf or something." Hugh imitates the therapist's voice, " 'Okay, concentrate now and throw the beanbag into the basket I'm holding.' He's holding a big plastic clothes hamper, pretending it's a basketball hoop, and shouting from a few feet away. I tried and missed. He yelled again, 'C'mon, Hugh, use your *left* hand. You can do better than that!' He lifted the hamper higher, and he was pissing me off.

'Concentrate hard and throw!' he yelled again. People were watching. I felt totally stupid. I made a decision. I concentrated with all my might, but not on the basket, on the guy's nose." Hugh laughs out loud.

"Did you hit him?" I ask.

"Yup! I lobbed it right in his face. I heard the other patients laughing."

"Hugh, that's awful!" I can't help smiling at how happy this makes him.

"You should have seen the guy yelling, 'No! Aim for the basket!' I guess it was rotten but it sure felt good!"

Hugh hasn't had the upper hand in a long time and he's pumped about this encounter. "You're too much!" I say. "But go easy on the poor guy tomorrow. Will you?" Although these sessions irritate Hugh, I begin to see a marked difference in his ability to focus. The Metronome therapy is working.

I spend a lot of time informing everyone about Hugh's impending plans to return to work. There are doctors, insurance companies, therapists, and disability insurance people to notify. Things are happening fast. Dr. G also wants Tom to meet Hugh's two speech therapists, Cathy and Michaelle, so he will be knowledgeable about brain injury and Hugh's problem areas.

Within days, Tom meets Cathy and begins his crash course in brain injury. I secretly wonder if Tom will withdraw his offer after hearing about the challenges Hugh will face.

Five days later, at a morning team meeting at HealthSouth, all reports are positive and upbeat. Metronome therapy is declared over. Hugh is given the go ahead to mow the lawn using his John Deere tractor. He is showered with encouragement for his return to work efforts, and we talk about coping and compensatory strategies. Michaelle warns him, "Look out for cognitive fatigue. Be sure to take short mental breaks to maintain your focus, and if you feel very tired, take a short rest."

Anxious to return to work, Hugh comes home from rehab, showers and puts on his business clothes. I drop him off at one p.m. and pick him up at five.

"How did it go?" I ask him.

"Well, I went to a few meetings and I think it's going okay," he says. As soon as he's in the front door, he darts upstairs.

"Where are you going?" I ask.

"To change, so I can mow the lawn," he says happily. Within minutes he's riding his tractor. I watch him through the kitchen window carving circles in the lawn as joyfully as if he's test-driving a new sports car.

Hugh works only two days his first week starting October 8th and three alternate mornings the following week. Work is challenging and he's worn out when he comes home. "There are so many deadlines," he tells me. "I feel disconnected because I'm not around enough. Don't forget, they have meetings when I'm not there, so I'm never sure what I've missed. And there's a new software system being implemented that I need to learn."

Demands are being made, demands with timelines and consequences. "Well, Hugh, this is an executive job," I say.

He nods. "I know," he says. But his face is lined with worry.

Our long-term disability case manager locates two job coaches to work with Hugh, but first they must test him to identify his needs. The test, which measures brain function, is called a neuropsychological exam. It takes seven hours to perform. The first available appointment for this test is not until October 30th, which means that Hugh will be at work for four weeks before the job coaches have the information necessary to create compensatory strategies for him. He's on his own at the most crucial time of his re-entry to work with no support system in place.

How did we let this happen? It all sounded so good just a short time ago.

Chapter 35

A Celebration of Friendship on October 19, 2002
You are invited to join us for a backyard party in your honor
For your friendship, sincerity, and help
For taking care of our house and making repairs,
For driving, cooking, praying, massaging, and mowing!
Please come dressed to play, laugh and relax at the Rawlins' house,

Six months out

The leaves in Virginia fall later than they do up north. In early October our backyard glints like fired charcoals in red, yellow and orange, but the leaves still cling to the branches and hang on in the breeze.

On a cool evening, I'm sitting at my computer desk in the front office. Mary walks over and leans in the doorjamb. "Hey Mom, what did Bambi leave on the front door yesterday?"

Looking up from the screen I answer, "Some pictures she took of you and Harley. They're on the kitchen counter." As she walks away, I hear her say, "Bambi is the most thoughtful person."

Within seconds, Anna strolls into my office and flops into the rocking chair. "Everyone's been really great to us. We have the best friends."

"We really do," I say. Mary returns and begins flipping through pictures, half-listening to us. I swivel my chair around when I hear the rocking chair creak. Mary has squeezed in beside Anna. They look at each other as Mary says, "Did we ever tell you that Patty King came over once when you weren't home and cleaned the house with us? She didn't want you to know she did it. It was so funny. We all rushed around cleaning and stuff. She's hilarious!"

"Are you kidding?" I ask with a short laugh. Then Anna chimes in, "Remember that huge hamper full of snacks from Dad's office? I think we ate those snacks for two months."

"And the quilted pillows Diana Stone made for us in the hospital." We could all feel an idea forming.

"And Barbara Farley, she came to the ICU, took you out to lunch, and she cooked us all that big delicious dinner. And don't forget the beautiful earrings Mrs. Young gave you just to cheer you up," Mary adds.

"Let's write it all down and send everyone thank you letters," I suggest. The girls start calling names out too fast for me to type. The list keeps growing. People visited, prayed, cooked, drove, cleaned, mowed, raked, and gave gifts, time, and food. I type until my fingers cramp up.

"Wait, let's just throw a party!" Mary screams as she jumps out of the chair. Anna joins in. "Yeah, Mom, a party would be so much fun!" she says. "Let's go get Dad." A few minutes later, after the sound of much scampering upstairs, a bewildered Hugh is led into the office.

"Look, Dad, look at this list of everyone that has helped us. We want to have a thank-you party. Can we?" Anna asks. Hugh leans into the computer and starts reading. Sweetness takes over his face, "Sure... Wow... look at that," he whispers.

"We'll make a banner," I propose. "We can blow it up at Kinko's and hang it up at the party. This will be so much fun!" The next few hours are spent thinking of every person that helped us along the way. When all is said and done, we ask about a hundred people over for a big informal outdoor gathering.

The Monday before the party, Hugh works morning hours for the first time. Tom picks him up early, as promised. In the afternoon, Hugh visits Dr. Ward who says he does not need to see him again for a year.

Hugh continues to juggle work with his rehab visits. From what he is telling me, he spends a lot of time trying to track down information in the office. He mentions meetings, but doesn't go into detail. He's only there a few hours a day, a few days a week, so it's hard to make an impact. His work coaches cannot help him until his neuropsych evaluation results are in, and the test has not even been conducted yet. Feeling both hopeful and ominous, I wonder: can a hundred friends cushion the blow if this job doesn't work out?

On the day of the party, our house comes alive with laughter and celebration. Friends and relatives pour in from as far away as California. Buckets of cold drinks dot the lawn. A lively volleyball game dominates the side of the house. Patty King sets out a buffet with Mom and they work together in the kitchen to keep the food trays filled. Pop delights the kids by wearing a balloon hat like the big kid he is. Everyone pauses to read the six-foot thank-you banner in the dining room, seeking out his or her own name among the helpers. After dark, my sister Peg tells stories about Hollywood to a group of teenagers in the living room while others congregate on the cool deck outside. Hugh soaks it all in—he's the center—the reason they came.

When the last of our friends have gone, a nagging thought keeps picking at my brain.

Tom, Hugh's boss, did not come to the party.

Chapter 36

*I ask only that you view me with an open mind,
and know that possibilities lie ahead for me.*

-Hugh

Seven months out

In an effort to sound casual, I ask, "Hugh, did Tom say he couldn't make it to the party for any reason? Did he have other plans?"

"None that I know of," he answers. It is not a good sign. I imagine Tom is distancing himself from us on a personal basis—it would be hard to go to a party with us, and then have to tell Hugh bad news. On Monday, Hugh wakes up early and Tom picks him up for work, as promised. I brace myself to deal with another disappointment, hoping my instincts are wrong.

When Hugh's work hours are over, I pick him up. He buckles his seatbelt and looks out the window—not at me. When I ask him what's wrong, he says, "Well, let me put it this way, Tom gave me the kind of talking to I've heard him give to other people when he was planning to let them go." I remain silent. Hugh continues, "Something's different about the way he's acting toward me. He asked me when I could add more hours."

"Isn't that a bit unreasonable?" I ask. "You've only been back to work five days. I know they haven't been consecutive, but it's not like he went into this with his eyes closed."

Hugh says nothing, so I continue. "I don't think anyone could meet Tom's expectations in twelve hours a week. You sometimes worked twelve hours in one day before your accident. Why did we agree to this?" I could kick myself for not listening to Dr. G.

"Yeah," Hugh says. "And the job coach wasn't there today. She couldn't make it in." I can hear the strain in his lowered voice.

Once home, I call the job coaches and mention Hugh's stress level at work. Both of them agree to see what they can do to help him cope and create realistic goals. Hugh tells me that Tom has set up weekly meetings with him to review what he has accomplished each week. Tom gave Hugh a spreadsheet of "Commitments and Expectations; not just goals" that dates back to June 2002. There are numerous objectives to achieve. Why are these goals still not met when it's now October? Why is it Hugh's job to fix old problems? I find myself feeling defensive, but behind my feelings, I understand the company's dilemma. Hugh always says, "Business is business."

One job coach tells me she's amazed at what Hugh has been able to do in such a short time. She says he is an admired leader, well respected by his managers and staff. I find it interesting that she thinks Hugh is doing so well. I doubt she's ever had to coach an employee at this high level. Plus, she has the TBI perspective—she sees what Hugh can accomplish *in spite* of his lingering deficits. She has seen others with his type of injury unable to perform at this level after many years. Tom, on the other hand, naturally compares Hugh to his former self, a high-achieving executive who gets results fast. He needs the "old" Hugh back. Tom can hardly be faulted for this; he's been trying to cover Hugh's workload for months now. Top management is shifting, and Tom's own position could be at stake. He needs help fast.

We've come so far. I try to convince myself that it is just a minor setback, something we had been warned about. There will be other jobs, other days, and other opportunities. I have to keep Hugh's spirits up. He has to keep trying. I think of ways I can frame this so he will understand that he is still moving forward, that this is not a giant step back. Why does it have to feel like such a loss?

The Friday meeting with Tom goes well, according to Hugh and his coach. Hugh addresses all of Tom's outstanding issues. He has met with people, and gotten the ball rolling on several initiatives. Hugh shares the status of all the tasks on his list; of course, the status is incomplete in many areas given the time he spends in the office. The job coach comes away from the meeting elated; she says all is well and on track. Again, I have a sense that the truth is being evaded. Hugh's coach is not a trained financial accounting executive. How can she assess his performance accurately?

Hugh isn't one to whine and make excuses, but I can see his discouragement in the creases of his eyes, his drooping head, and defeated shoulders. In the past, when stress piled up, he could get on his bike and ride thirty miles to recharge. Now, there is no road stretched out before him; the road is off limits. The garage is a lonely place. The wind-trainer leads nowhere.

When we walk, I keep talking to him about new beginnings. Returning to his former position is not the only option; it is a job, plain and simple. Jobs change, life changes, but the important things remain with us if we let them: family, relationships, and health. We begin talking about change.

Hugh's subsequent Friday meetings with Tom are over quickly. There is little feedback and Hugh says he feels invisible. Tom's demeanor is cordial but strained. Because there is no direct negative feedback, no one sees the train wreck ahead, but Hugh and I can hear the rumbling in the distance.

On October 30th, Hugh completes a neuropsychological exam administered by MCV's renowned Jeff Kreutzer. The exam is comprised of a series of tests designed to measure individual aspects of Hugh's brain function. Prior to testing, they determined Hugh's pre-injury function by using several tools: his résumé, job description, educational level, and questionnaires. They rated him against the general population as either above average, average, low average, borderline impaired or impaired. It is determined that Hugh had been above average in nearly all areas pre-injury, so it is explained to us that significant changes in functional ability below that marker suggest lingering effects of the brain injury.

We spend seven hours at MCV. I participate in the first part of the information-gathering session, completing a questionnaire and answering some questions. After that, Hugh takes the tests alone until noon with an hour break for lunch followed by three more hours of testing. By three p.m., he's done. "My brain is fried," he says, as he limps along to the car exhausted. He has spent every last cell remembering, sorting, and figuring.

Once home, HealthSouth calls to say Hugh is being released from physical and occupational therapy. His official release from the day program is set for November 5th. He will then transfer to outpatient therapy to continue speech/cognitive work. Knowing how athletic Hugh has always been, I urge him to continue working out on his own at our gym. I'm convinced that exercise helps his brain. Since my work schedule is flexible, I can drop him off some afternoons to do upper body exercises on his own.

The following week, he starts training at American Family Fitness. While he's working out, I meet a résumé client. After my meeting, I'm a little early to pick him up, so I park and go inside. In a huge room full of exercise equipment I see Hugh wandering from one machine to another, looking dazed. His gait is aimless, and his left arm flops the way it did before his final surgery. He sees me, offers a pathetic half-smile, but his eyes are clouded in sadness. On the way home I ask him, "What's bothering you?"

"I feel like I'm waiting for the other shoe to drop," he says. I remember what the nurse practitioner told me before his last surgery: "Stress often manifests itself physically after a TBI." I can see the stress flattening him like a monstrous demolition machine.

"What is making you feel this way?" I ask. His face is turned away from me, looking out the window, his temple leaning on the headrest.

"The other morning, when Tom drove me to work and we got out of the car, he looked annoyed. He's made some comments. I can't please him. I know he's thinking of letting me go."

"Hugh, I don't think he's angry with you as much as he's angry with the situation. He's stuck with a very hard choice and he considers you a friend. But the truth is: he may have to let you go, so he's putting on a hard shell. He needs more help than you can give him now."

Hugh takes it hard. Tom is obviously frustrated and Hugh feels like the cause of it. He acutely senses that things are different. I tell him to discuss it with Michaelle at rehab and he does. Michaelle makes him feel a little better. "Hugh," she says, "Don't let Tom's attitude bother you. Look, the guy has no idea what you've been through. No one does but you. Use this job as therapy and take what you can for yourself."

This advice is easier said than done. Hugh hates to fail, and this feels like a huge personal failure to him. Usually he can take steps to correct a situation, but he can't fix this problem—the tools don't work right yet. This profound sense of failure is exactly what Dr. G wanted to avoid.

Hugh's sadness disturbs me, so I call our vocational rehab counselor at the insurance company. She makes a phone call to Tom and asks him directly if Hugh's return to work plan is succeeding. Later she tells me that Tom said things haven't worked out the way he thought they would. She told Tom he had to be honest with Hugh. It would be unfair to drag things out.

At a meeting on November 8th, Tom tells Hugh and the job coaches that he needs to hire a new Assistant Controller. He says he needs someone who can work forty to sixty hours a week and take over his job, if need be. Hugh later tells me that Tom said, "There's no one right now that can fill the shoes that Hugh once wore. Before his injury, Hugh was the one person I could have relied upon to take over. It's just not the case anymore."

"It made me feel both proud and sad at the same time," Hugh says.

I imagine that Tom has grappled with this for weeks and finally realized what a brain injury is: a complicated change in a person that is not fully apparent at first glance.

"Tom asked me to think about how I can add value to the corporation in another area and says he will work with me to try another job that may work out better," Hugh says.

"Well it sounds like he wants to make things up to you," I say.

"Sounds like a demotion to me."

Hugh says little else. The next morning, he asks me to drive him to the gym so he can work out. Anna and I drop him off, run errands, and return to pick him up. When he throws his gear in the car, he appears frazzled. Out of nowhere, he laughs the way someone laughs when they have had too much bad luck.

"Did anything happen while you worked out?" I ask.

"Kind of. I locked my gym bag, keys, and cell phone in my locker and went to warm up on the rowing machine. A little while later, I went to get my basketball sneakers, but I couldn't remember which locker I used."

"Oh No!" says Anna. "What did you do, Dad?"

"Well, my lock is the old one you kept on your school locker, the simple, silver type. Trouble was... the same one was on just about every locker in there. I knew the combination, so I decided I'd just start trying a few in the general vicinity to see if I got lucky. Then I noticed suspicious looks from naked guys wondering if I was a thief. One guy looked mad, so I left the locker room."

"What happened?" I pressed.

"I walked to the front desk and asked the receptionist to call my cell phone number so I could hear my locker ring. Then I ran back to the locker room and it worked! But then I still couldn't get the combination to open it, so the maintenance man had to cut the lock off." Hugh laughs.

Anna's mouth is agape. She laughs and says, "Dad, that's embarrassing! I'm never going to the gym with you again!"

"Have you thought any more about the job?" I ask.

"Not much to think about. Tom is putting an ad in the paper next week for my replacement, but I still supposedly have a job...still getting paid. It's just weird."

"Well, just hang in there till we will get the results of the neuropsych evaluation. That should help us decide what to do," I say. "I'm glad you're working out again."

"Yeah, I need a new lock. Can you get one that has a wild design on it so I can tell which one is mine?" he suggests. Once home, I email Tom and tell him I'll drive Hugh to work from now on if he can come to work at eight in the morning instead of earlier. Everyone is more comfortable with this new arrangement.

By midweek, Tom has drafted a new job for Hugh. It is a few pay scales lower and involves Hugh working *under* managers who used to report to him.

There is also a caveat in the offer: Hugh has to prove he will be "adding value" in his new position. But the definition of "adding value" is not all that clear. Hugh says he thinks this takes away from the spirit in which the offer is being made.

While filling me in, Hugh says, "I asked Tom, 'What would you do if you were me?' and he told me he wouldn't take it. It would hurt his pride too much. At least he was honest."

As we wait for the neuropsychological test results, Hugh has long discussions with his therapists and several close friends.

Nancy Foley has been away having foot surgery for a few weeks, but has now returned to work. As we sit in her office looking a bit sullen, she says, "Well, the way I see the situation is this: If you accept the lower position offered, Hugh, you will have blurred boundaries with the people who used to report to you. There may be more feelings of discomfort, just as you've experienced with Tom. In addition, there is always the possibility of anything going wrong being blamed on you, not intentionally, but because they may now associate any mistake as resulting from the brain injury. You can easily wind up a scapegoat."

Hugh and I nod in agreement. It is hard news to hear. Nancy goes on. "But there could be an upside. If you feel comfortable doing this, you could retain a position in the company and work toward a promotion in the future. It will take some serious thinking."

We also discuss Hugh's ongoing recovery. The landscape of his brain is improving on a daily basis. Sometimes the changes are so dramatic you can see them day-to-day, like the day he tied his shoes, or when he simply started getting up in the morning on time. Other changes are subtle, like his speed of processing. Nancy's concern is that judgments will be made and opinions set before Hugh is at his peak. In her comforting way, Nancy encourages us to explore other possibilities before making the decision, and one is to simply let Hugh get the rest he desperately needs in a stress-free environment before returning to any level of work. This had been Dr. G's recommendation from the start.

This transition week, as we try to find a direction, is grueling to say the least. Our caseworker from the long-term insurance company calls and says, "I'm just so sorry you and Hugh had to go through the meat grinder. It was really way too soon for him to attempt this." I see more and more how the world now seems divided in two: those who understand brain injury and those who don't. Society, as a whole, and the legal system do not understand the lifelong effects of TBI, nor do they want to pay for them. Once a person begins to look better, it's assumed he is well. This injury has the potential to sabotage frequent return-to-work efforts and not even be acknowledged as the cause of his inability to perform, once he is released from medical care. There is a serious lack of knowledge about it in the general public, and that lack of knowledge leads to grim consequences for TBI patients and their families.

Our lifeline is our friends, family, and the professionals who understand the story from beginning to end. This is an exhausting story to live, no less recount. My friends continue to sustain me. Without their listening ears and understanding hearts, I would have never been able to support Hugh so well. Hugh's friends keep him busy on weekends and with phone calls. Many of his friendships have been transformed. Some friends have faded away while other connections have deepened. Instead of just riding bikes and joking superficially, he and his friends talk about their families, life plans, and feelings. Walking, running, eating out, and going to ball games have become activities they enjoy together, not just cycling.

As the days grow shorter and colder, we begin pulling out our winter clothes. Hugh owns a bright red sweater that is a favorite of mine. I always tell him he looks handsome in it. One morning, as he is dressing in our bedroom, there is a knock on the door. He calls, "Come in," and sees Mary. She stares at him in astonishment. His wide shoulders are scrunched into her small red tent dress with the wide navy umpire stripe nearly reaching his throat; his arms and chest are bursting the seams open. He is wearing it like a shirt with his blue jeans. "Dad, why are you wearing my red dress?" she asks.

"I'm not. This is my red sweater. Your mom told me she liked it on me."

"No, Dad, that's my dress." He steps over to the mirror and takes a look, "But it was hanging in my closet," he says, lamely.

Mary turns and says, "Let's go ask Mom." The two of them walk down the stairs. Anna and I are in the kitchen. We look at Hugh, then at each other.

"Isn't that Mary's red dress you're wearing?" I ask.

He looks surprised, "I am? I thought it was a little tight." We all stand motionless for a moment, holding our breath. Hugh lets out a chuckle, starting a chain reaction of hysterical laughter. Anna screams out between snorts, "Dad, I can't believe you're wearing Mary's dress!" The girls jump around him, offering hugs of playfulness.

"Sorry Hon, this is partly my fault. I hung it there to remind myself to take it to Goodwill. I'll be more careful about what I hang on your side of the closet!" I say.

We're still not sure if he should accept the new job offer. On Friday we attend the team meeting with Dr. Kreutzer, the two job coaches, Liz West (our lawyer), and Michaelle (Hugh's speech therapist). Only Dr. Kreutzer has seen the report. As in all team meetings, we've come to find, there is bad news to be delivered with the good, and it is not easy to do it eloquently, but Dr. Kreutzer is a pure professional.

The meeting begins. Dr. Kreutzer points to some marked deficits, and Michaelle agrees they match her assessments over the past several months. Sustained attention and concentration continue to be problems. Hugh's general fund of information is found to be within the low average range and arithmetic calculation skills in the average range, but below expectations. On a positive note, his reading has improved to the 86th percentile. His common sense and safety reasoning rank very high. Since Hugh was rated *above average* before the injury, many scores are not in that range, and there are some shocking impairments that persist, most relating to the executive function areas: initiation, organization, planning, and information processing rate. Stamina is also a lingering problem. The room is thick with reflection, everyone cocooned in their own thoughtful space, knowing how hard this must be for Hugh to hear and process, especially in the presence of a group.

Hugh feels the uneasiness and wants no part of it. He breaks the tension with an occasional funny remark. In a strange way, he is the leader of this group, showing us he knows everyone is rooting for him, for his best interest, bad news or good. I'm sure he feels like doubling over or running away, but he soothes us with his acceptance of the facts, his ability to absorb successive blows. I hold back my tears in the meeting, my throat clogged with the ache of his courage in the face of hardship.

Dr. Kreutzer looks thoughtfully around the table before resting his eyes on Hugh. "Take some time to grieve for your old life," he says, and pauses to let the words sink in. Continuing gently he adds, "Many people want to go back to the life they had before, but this is not possible for most people. In general, it takes three to five years for people to find their way after trial and error, but most do, and with a good deal of happiness in the end." Hugh and I flinch. Three to five YEARS?

Seeing our expressions, the doctor continues, "Five percent of people with Hugh's severity of injury are confined to a nursing home and cannot feed themselves. Hugh, you are on the high-functioning end of the spectrum for your severity of brain injury. You are quite remarkable."

Grieve for your old life.

The words hover above my consciousness before meaning sears into me. Time frames reverberate in my head: in three months he'll have made the most progress, maybe six months, a year, progress even after two years or longer.

Is our old life gone?

Forever?

What can this mean? Can he hold down a job again? Will he ever drive a car? Can he be active and happy again? When he asks, "When will I be normal?" is the answer: never?

NO! The word rips through my head. Something in me shouts he'll get better. After all, he had only a ten percent chance to live, and he's taken a rigorous test, he's attempted a demanding executive job. He failed because it was too soon. Am I blind? Am I not willing to face the truth?

We return home to a ringing phone and the voice of Michaelle, his speech therapist. She urges Hugh not to be discouraged. The news is good. Hugh is on the path to recovery and it just takes time. She catches the door just before it slams for good when she reminds him that this is a six-month assessment; things will surely improve by twelve months. We spend two hours in a paralyzing stupor, digesting all this new information.

Reflecting on the first family meeting at MCV, I remind Hugh of the incredible strides he has made. He could read only three words just five months ago and is now above average in reading. He has read an entire book in two days and discussed it intelligently with me. "Michaelle is right, Hugh. You are not done healing. There's so much more to do. You can do this."

It's late Friday afternoon and the girls burst in the front door eager for the weekend. Their presence immediately animates the room, filling it with energy. We gaze at them, their once-steady parents now teetering on the edge. A voice inside me commands, "Find your footing, find it fast." Hugh is looking past the girls, his eyes staring into some unknown place.

I had been forewarned that depression is almost inevitable following brain injury, and from the stories I heard, I feel certain that depression is what often stalls recovery. I decide to attack it head on and help Hugh fight it. "Hugh, we'll work together and take our time to do things right. We can't fall into the pit. We'll figure it out." After more talk about the offer his company has made, we draft a letter dated November 25, 2002.

Dear Tom,

I have decided to decline the offer of Accountant 2 and take more time to recover, as strongly suggested by my physician.

In recent discussions with you I asked, "Would this demotion job change negatively impact my future at this company and other places?" After much thought, I have come to realize that the answer to that question is, undoubtedly, "Yes."

We have had lengthy discussions regarding brain injury before I decided to take my "scaled back Assistant Controller" position. You proposed that I try eight weeks working three days a week, 4 hours a day, then gradually increase those hours as the doctor approved and I further recuperated. While I understand that the demands of this position require someone who can stay in the loop and be able to work 40-60 hours a week, I was also up front about what I could and could not do before coming back to work.

We also thoroughly discussed the nature of brain injury with Rosemary (my wife), my therapists, the LTD Coordinator, and job coaches – I am in the PROCESS of recovery. While I am not yet where I use to be, I am continually improving and building stamina. Therefore, with the right hours, coaching and mentoring, it is entirely possible that I could return to my former status at some point in the future somewhere. Should I compromise that by returning to a company in a much lower position where everyone who does not know that I am continually improving will think this is the end result of the injury? It does not make sense to do_that. It's in my best interest, and in the interest of the company, that I return to disability status to recover further; and possibly apply for available positions at a later date.

I would like to keep the door open. As a highly productive, well-respected employee, I think that is a reasonable expectation for the future. I ask only that you view me with an open mind and know that possibilities lie ahead for me. I have worked very hard to come this far and will continue to push myself to be the best that I can be.

I would like to take this opportunity to thank you all for the time, patience and support you have offered my family and me during this very difficult period in my life, especially, Kelly, Dixie and Michelle, in the last several weeks. It has meant a lot to all of us.

Hugh

Chapter 37

Dear Rosie, Hugh, Anna and Mary,
Know you are in my thoughts and prayers daily. You have a tough road ahead of
you, but I know you have the strength and love to see this through to a brighter
side. Yes, there is sadness, but we as a family have found a great closeness and
spirit within that brings rays of light and laughter too. Please know that I'm
there for you all in spirit.
Hugs and kisses all around with lots of love always,
KiKi, Tom, Thomas, Drew and Erin

        -My cousin, KiKi Doherty, New York

Seven months out

Hugh sits at the kitchen table pretending to read the paper. Looking up, he says out of nowhere, "What am I supposed to do now? Sometimes I'm not sure I know who I am anymore."

"You're who you always were—a man with a loving family and tons of friends. A hundred friends came to your party, remember? You have choices now. You can try new things," I say.

"What if I just want my old job back? That's not a choice."

"Well Hon, we both know you're still getting better. Maybe some-day you will have a job just like your old job. We just have to wait and see."

He looks back down at the newspaper. I can see my answers don't satisfy him.

When I email the Lance Armstrong Foundation, an organization devoted to cancer victims and their families, I reach a woman named Sally, a cancer survivor herself. We never meet, and yet we email back and forth and she reaches out to me in a profound way. I ask her in desperation, "How can I help my husband? I feel so useless. What can I do to make a difference?"

She writes back: "Remind him that you love him. Remind him of his past. Remind him that you love him. Remind him of your history with each other. Remind him of his daughters' birthdays, your birthday, anniversary, and remind him that you love him. Talk to him, talk to him, talk to him, and remind him."

I want Hugh to know I still believe in our marriage, that I believe in him. I want a deep commitment, a future. I am not staying with him out of pity or a sense of obligation. I stay with him because he's my life partner, because I can't imagine living without him.

As we walk around our neighborhood, wearing a familiar path up Joseph Drive, past the row of newly vinyl-sided houses and manicured lawns, I try again to connect. "We have to let go of the work labels that we think define us, and look at the relationships that make up our lives. You are more than an assistant controller; you're a father, a friend, a son, and a husband. These are the things I love about you. Your job is just a job. They come and go."

Hugh exhales a white puff in the evening chill. He looks skeptical. "I worked all my life to get to where I was in that job. It's a lot to let go of. It's hard to feel worth much without it. Being a father, husband, and friend doesn't put dinner on the table." His head droops.

When I squeeze his hand hard he looks at me while I say, "I know. I am proud of what you achieved at work. But I'm even prouder of what you have achieved since your accident. You have fought hard to come back to us. There must be a reason for that. It wasn't so you could work long hours at the office."

"Still, I can't work. I can't surf or ride my bike with the guys. I can't drive the girls around..." his grip weakens.

"Not yet, but you will. You'll get your license back. Think of it this way, you are still putting dinner on the table through the insurance coverage you have. The insurance coverage you *earned* and are using legitimately. When we first met, we knew nothing about each other.

There was just that initial connection, that attraction, that feeling that drew us together. Those things are still there, regardless of what we do or where we work. We always have each other. The other things are accessories. What I guess I'm trying to say is, I love you without the accessories."

"But what about those other things I can't do. The things I used to love doing. The sports..." his voice trails off, almost breaking.

"No one is saying you will never do them again. Just not for the time being, until you get a little better. I know it's hard to wait. But in the meantime let's enjoy life together; enjoy what we do have right now. I am thankful for this, to just have you here." He manages a fragile smile, but he is not convinced. His sadness weighs heavily on me.

Thanksgiving comes in the same week as Hugh formally leaves his job for good. His last day is like the final body blow in a long round of boxing, the concrete evidence that this accident has indeed changed his life. But, after a few days of hiding under the covers, talking a lot and rediscovering what it is to start over once again, we begin to look forward.

We take long walks and Hugh goes jogging for forty minutes alone one afternoon. When he comes in the front door breathless after his workout, he is drenched in sweat and clearly invigorated. I hand him a glass of water and can barely contain my smile.

"Hugh, did you know your shorts are inside out?"

"No," he laughs. "At least I'm not wearing a red dress."

Later, I watch him work in the yard. He's cutting down brush that has overgrown and raking the last of the fall leaves. Physical activity helps his mood.

One chilly afternoon he returns to his home office, and in a frenzy of cleaning, he fills three brown grocery bags with discarded papers. We talk about our future. "I'll bag groceries if I have to—for you and the girls. I'll flip burgers," he says. "It's not like I ever looked down on any kind of work. I think all work is good if people do it for the right reasons. I want you and the girls to be happy."

"I can help too," I say. "I did work a corporate job for twelve years before we had the girls, remember? For now, we're fine. We're managing."

Our family of four spends Thanksgiving alone. We pass on an invitation to Rhode Island to spend the weekend with my sister and parents; the trip seems too long and arduous after the draining previous weeks. Instead, we visit Electra and meet her extended Greek family in the morning. Hugh goes for a run around the neighborhood wearing the blue knit cap Bambi made him. The girls rattle pots and prepare dishes as we play loud music in the kitchen. Clad in flannel pajama pants and thin-strapped dance tops, they peel, chop, mix and stir, in the warm herb-scented corner by the stove. The smalls of their backs are exposed as they sway to music in bare feet while they work.

Before dinner, we join hands around the candlelit table in prayer and bless those near and far whom we love. When the time comes for Hugh to say what he is thankful for, his eyes fill up with tears. He chokes out the words, "All my girls." He weeps openly. The girls let out nervous laughs and pat his arm. They roll their eyes. "I'm sorry," he sniffles.

A friend had recently asked me, "What's it like having Hugh with a different personality?"

"Well...it's the best of both worlds," I said. "It's like I'm having an affair without having to cheat on my husband."

Hugh is still himself in many ways. It's not just the injury that has changed him. It's the overwhelming expressions of love and support he's received that have also changed him. He's like Ebenezer Scrooge; he's traveled with the Ghost of Christmas Yet to Come. He's been able to see the impact his life has had on others because he came so close to the end. It's humbling, and it fills him up.

Chapter 38

There really is a Santa!

Eight months out

The holidays are approaching. Hugh glances at the calendar on his office wall—the empty boxes remind him that he has nothing to look forward to. "There's plenty to do around here," I point out, while dumping a basket of laundry on the bed. I stare at him as I begin folding. He raises his eyebrows and smirks.

Hugh needs options now, something active. Dr. Kreutzer recommends volunteer work, but that has no appeal to him yet. I suspect he's battling depression. Cold days and harsh rains prevent him from running as often as he wants. He's forced to spend time resting, reading, and working through his sense of loss internally.

I continue my writing. Pouring out my feelings on paper becomes my therapy. "Maybe you should take up writing," I suggest.

"I think not," he says. "I'm the numbers guy, remember?"

"Maybe you'd surprise yourself. It feels good to bang words out on the computer and make them disappear with one touch of a key—too bad there's not a delete key for the problems in our lives."

Dr. Kreutzer has been helping us plan our "new life." One of Hugh's first questions is direct. "Do you think I'll ever be a CFO?" he asks. It's a career goal he's had for years now.

"Not for at least five to ten years," says the doctor. I suspect he doesn't even think that will be possible, but he is a smart enough man to avoid dashing Hugh's hopes completely. "For now, I think it's best to concentrate on being a couple and help each other at home. Take it slow," the doctor suggests.

One night after dinner, I ask Hugh if he will do the dishes. I'm beginning to think that maybe he should do more around the house, especially if I have to go back to work full-time at some point. "Later," he says while slumping in his recliner to watch television. An hour goes by, so I ask again, "Hugh, are you going to wash the dishes or not?"

"I said I'd do it later," he says, annoyed. I leave the room in a huff and scrub the dishes myself. At bedtime, Hugh is apologetic. "I don't want to lose you and the girls," he says, more upset than he should be over the incident. "Sometimes I think you would all have been better off if I had died in that accident."

"Absolutely not! Hugh, nothing would be worse than that."

"Oh really? Living with a loser isn't worse?"

"You're not a loser, you're getting better. Promise me you will never ever do anything to hurt yourself! Nothing! Nothing would hurt the girls or me more than losing you that way. It would not help us; it would devastate us. Maybe you should talk to…"

"Don't worry," he cuts in, "that would be a permanent solution to a short term problem. I wouldn't do that to you. I just sometimes wonder why I made it." He pulls me close and kisses my cheek.

"Then why did you say that? Really Hugh, this is serious…"

"I mean it. I would never do that to you and the girls. Hey, next time I'll wash the dishes too," he says.

"Well, you *did* make me forget about the stupid dishes," I say elbowing him with a loud sniff. "Way to change the subject!" When he smiles, I add, "Hey, maybe it's good we're fighting over dirty dishes now. Doesn't that feel so ordinary?"

"Yeah, only I thought we were fighting over suicide!"

"You're morbid! Stop…"

"You talk too much, do you know that?" he says, kissing me again.

"I love you," I whisper.

"You better," he says, and he dozes off. I stare at him as he sleeps, jealous. Sleep never sneaks up on me anymore.

Hugh continues to recuperate into the winter months. We take long walks and talk every evening. Day by day he's able to stay awake longer, while still maintaining attention. He's working on the computer again. I send him emails, articles to read, and links to follow, and anxiously await notes back from him.

The week before Christmas, Hugh takes on the project of assembling a small bicycle with training wheels for a friend's son. He feels a sense of accomplishment when the last bolt is secured.

On Christmas Eve, we attend the midnight candlelight service at church. On our return home, we find a beautiful holiday basket on our front porch that contains several generous gift certificates. All certificates are signed "Santa." We have no idea who left them. "There really is a Santa," Anna and Mary shout, as they link arms in the kitchen and dance around.

Staring out the back window, my imagination sees a sleigh and reindeer arching across the sky. "Thank-you" I whisper. People are so good.

Chapter 39

Diary Entry:
Happy New Year! Glad 2002 is over!

Nine months out

January 14th is a momentous day! Hugh passes his driving evaluation through HealthSouth and regains his right to drive. "Hey, let's celebrate. I'll take you for a spin!" he says.

"Okay. Go slow. Hugh, the red light!" I shriek as I grip the handle above the car door tight enough for a one-armed pull-up.

"I see it," he says calmly. He's soaking in the experience of the car, the feel of the steering wheel, the sun that shines through the closed window warming the side of his face.

"Try not to tailgate!" My feet press hard against the floor.

"Rosemary, would you relax?"

"I would if I could! Just be careful!" The first time he ventures out alone, I ask him to come back within an hour. "Please put up with my nerves for a little while," I beg him. "Once you drive a few times without any problems, I'll calm down."

He rolls his eyes at me, gives me a squeeze and says, "I understand." While he's out, I scour the bathrooms until my hands are raw. Exactly an hour later, the phone rings, making me jump.

"Hey!" It's Hugh's voice.

"Hugh? Where are you?"

"I am five minutes away, but I knew you'd be a basket case.

Everything's fine. I'll be right home." After a few days, I begin to enjoy the freedom Hugh's ability to drive affords me. He drives around and looks at properties, runs to the store, works out at the gym, and drops the girls at school when they need a ride. He walks taller and straighter. He even has a slight bounce in his step. "Now I'm going to buy you a car," he says proudly.

He drives all over town test driving and pricing vehicles, then takes me to see three cars he thinks I'll like. We purchase a nearly new Honda Accord. When my sister, Peg, hears the price, she says, "Now there's a job for him, he can be a professional car price negotiator. Damn he's good!"

In February, Hugh enrolls in a two-week real estate class to prepare for the state exam and hopefully a new career. "The classes are Monday through Friday from nine in the morning until four in the afternoon," I remind him. "Long hours. Sure you can do that?"

"Yup," he smiles. Michaelle, his speech/cognitive therapist from HealthSouth, gives him tips. "Make sure you rest when you're home, take frequent breaks. Take good notes and review often." Concerned that he's taking on too much too soon once again, she cautions against high expectations.

Hugh repeats his now familiar saying, "If it's to be, it's up to me."

Full of purpose, Hugh wakes happily in the morning. After class he darts out the front door for a run; if it's raining, he drives to the gym for a short workout. He is completely independent for the first time in nine months.

On Valentine's Day, Hugh has his first real estate test. The night before, he stays up late studying. It is a timed test to be completed within two and a half hours. Dr. Kreutzer advises that Hugh ask for extra time if he needs it. Hugh chooses not to ask and goes in at nine a.m. to start the exam. At eleven, I hear the front door creak open as I stand by the kitchen sink washing apples. I turn around and see Hugh walking toward me, his face half hidden by flowers. "Happy Valentine's Day," he says. "These are the ones, right?" He's holding a bouquet of alstroemeria, my favorite, and two bunches of pink carnations for the girls.

"How beautiful! Thank you!" I say with a kiss. "But what about the test? Did you finish? Was it hard?" I wipe off my hands and rummage through my lower cabinet for a few vases.

"I finished early. It was kind of tough," he says. "I just came home to have lunch with you. We'll get our grades this afternoon." We sit down to sandwiches and chips as he tells me about some of the questions on the test. Later in the afternoon when he arrives home, he's obviously pleased with himself. "I got an 84 on the test," he reports, with a sense of relief in his voice.

When Anna rushes in after school she sees Hugh sitting in his recliner. Out of breath, she unzips her coat, and asks, "Dad, how'd the test go?"

"I didn't get an A," he replies. He tells her his grade and she leans down to give him a big hug. "Next time, I'll study harder and I'll get an A," he mumbles with his face scrunched into the nape of her neck. She hugs him tighter. "I know you will, Dad."

The snow starts that night. A massive slow-moving East Coast storm blows in. We play Scrabble at the kitchen table and watch movies on TV while the snow piles up outside. The rich smell of roast chicken and hot bread fills the kitchen. Stuffed and satisfied, we snuggle into pillows and throw blankets on the couch, contentedly crowded in our own cozy nest.

On Sunday, church is cancelled due to the snowfall, now about seven inches deep. Monday and Tuesday, schools and classes are cancelled. The kitchen fills with the smell of cookies baking and the rich scent of thick hot chocolate and coffee.

"Tell me again why school is closed?" Hugh asks. "Can't people drive down here?"

"You know they don't have enough plows," I say.

"This would never happen in Vermont. You girls are spoiled," he says poking Anna's ribs.

"Then I'm glad we don't live in Vermont anymore!" Anna says, offering up a cookie.

By Wednesday, Hugh's real estate class is open, but the public schools are still closed because the back roads are not yet plowed. "This is ridiculous," Hugh mutters on his way out the door for his class. Later, he tells me the class was more challenging and covered extra material, so he reads and reviews all evening until his eyes are black underneath.

At bedtime, he can't settle down. He tosses, turns and gets out of bed a few times. In the morning, he confesses he was up until almost four a.m. By seven-thirty, he's ready to head out to class. "Be careful driving," I warn. "Call me if you feel too tired. Sure you're not too tired?"

"I'm fine!" At three o'clock, he walks in the front door, throws his book on the couch as though he's releasing a great burden, and let's out a long exhale.

"You're home early," I say, curious.

"The teacher cut it short so people who live far away could drive. These pansies are still afraid of the snow that's left. I think I'll go for a workout at the gym," he says.

"You must be overtired, Hon. Why don't you rest first," I suggest. I get a chill thinking of his driving when he hasn't slept much. He takes my advice, and attempts to nap in the recliner, but after an hour, he's restless. "I'm really not that tired. I'll just do a short workout and be home in plenty of time for dinner," he says leaving with his gym bag.

By five-thirty, I begin to worry, but I shrug it off as my usual over-attentiveness. I calm myself into being rational and tell myself he probably bumped into a friend or is taking a long, hot shower. While fixing dinner in the kitchen, the phone rings. Mary answers. "Mom, it's a fireman." She hands me the receiver with a twisted expression on her face.

"Mrs. Rawlins, this is Ed Wood from the Henrico Fire Department. Don't panic. Your husband is okay now. I'm with him at American Family. He had a seizure while working out."

Looking up from the phone, I quickly mouth to the girls, "Dad's okay."

"Did he fall and hit his head?" I ask.

"No, he was on the elliptical, but people around here say he stepped down off it, lowered himself to the ground then had a five to six minute seizure, probably a grand mal seizure. This is the same man I helped almost a year ago in the bike accident, isn't it?"

"Yes," I say, feeling sick.

"He's going to be all right, Ma'am. This is common with head injuries. It's a piece of cake compared to what he's already been through. I'll take him to Henrico Doctor's Hospital. It'll be closer for you than MCV."

"I'll leave right now and meet you there."

"Don't panic and don't rush, Mrs. Rawlins. He's in good hands. He seems to be remembering things. He's lucid. Take your time." The girls look more anxious each second.

"Thank you. I'll be there soon." Before I place the phone on the counter, Mary asks, "What happened?"

"Dad had a seizure at the gym. He's okay. He didn't hurt himself. I need to go to the hospital." I pick up a glass of water, start to drink it, and spill it all over the front of my shirt.

"Sure, you're okay, Mom," Anna says mockingly, trying to make light of the situation.

"Ed Wood was the rescue guy again," I say. "What are the chances of that happening?"

"That's weird, it's like he's Dad's guardian angel," Mary says.

We have a friend coming over at eight o'clock from out of town and have no hotel number to reach him, so Mary puts out an offer, "Mom, I'll stay here and tell Al what happened." Anna looks at me, "I'll come with you." They fall right in line.

"Mary, I don't want you here all alone…"

"I'll call Harley. Don't worry, I'm fine, Mom. Dad's gonna be fine too. Ed said so." She sounds ten years older than her age, more in control than I feel.

Hugh is reclining on a gurney in the ER, awake, but pale and sweaty when I arrive with Anna. Dressed in his wringing wet gym clothing, shorts, and a t-shirt, he smiles reassuringly as we enter the room. Ed Wood gives me a sideways hug. "It's been a hard year for you all, hasn't it?" he says. I nod in agreement.

The doctor walks in and informs us that Hugh needs a CAT scan to be sure there is nothing new going on because of his brain injury. After the test, they load him up with Dilantin. Hugh cannot seem to stand without his blood pressure dropping, so we wait. Finally, near midnight, he's stable and we leave the hospital with strict orders to see a neurologist right away.

Once home, I help Hugh into the house and up the stairs. We both fall into a deep sleep, glad to be in our own bed. Four hours later, in a half-sleep, I hear Hugh getting out of bed.

"Are you okay?" I ask groggily.

"I'm fine," he says. "Just going to the bathroom." I hear the door close lightly and the next minute I hear a thump. I run in and find him slumped over the toilet on his knees. As I grab him under the arms, Anna comes running in. I'm holding him up from behind, my arms around his chest. "Look at his face," I say. "Anna, is he awake? Hugh can you hear me?" No response.

"He's awake, Mom," she says.

"Hugh, can you stand up?" I ask.

"Yes," he says quietly, then proceeds to slip and slide on the vinyl bathroom floor like the scarecrow from *The Wizard of Oz.*

While holding Hugh, I say, "Get Dad a pillow." Anna runs into the bedroom and grabs a bed pillow, places it under his head and I gently slide him down. We settle blankets on him and he falls instantly asleep. Wide-awake now, Anna and I trudge downstairs and share a hot cup of tea. We take turns checking on Hugh every few minutes.

"You okay, Mom?" she asks.

"I'm fine, babe. You should go back to bed," I say. "And thank you." She hesitantly retreats to her room. After about thirty minutes I wake Hugh up to get him back into bed. Lying beside him, I rub his hair until he falls asleep. When I see the sun peeking through the shades, I give up trying to sleep, and sneak off the bed to make a pot of coffee.

Hugh needs food in his stomach after skipping dinner the night before and all the drugs at the hospital. As he downs an instant breakfast milkshake and muffin in bed, the color returns to his cheeks. When he shuffles into the shower, I decide to hang around like I used to and check on him. I speak to him through the fabric shower curtain.

"How are you doing?" I ask.

"I'm fine." His voice sounds far off. After a few minutes in the hot shower, with shampoo all over his head, I look in and see he is growing pale.

"Hugh?"

"I'm fine," he answers, but his body begins to sag. His eyelids slowly close. I step into the shower in my pajamas and hold him under the arms with water cascading all around us. He is half awake but faint. He slides to his knees, holding on to the shower seat while I rinse his head and help him out onto the bathroom floor, where he lies, wrapped in towels, while I dry off. Once his dizziness clears, I help him to the bed. He sleeps soundly until late morning. When he wakes up, he is much more himself. After he's dressed, I insist we use the gait belt to get downstairs. Just as Hugh settles into a kitchen chair, the doorbell rings. It's Lee Facetti with lunch for Hugh.

"Hey, how's it goin?" Lee yells as he kicks off his shoes by the front door. He pulls up a kitchen chair. "Rough night, huh?" He sits with us through a simple fast food meal and with his usual upbeat personality, tries to make us feel better. After eating, he chauffeurs me to American Family to pick up Hugh's Explorer, left in the parking lot the night before when the ambulance had come. In Lee's car, I vent, "This just plain stinks. He was beginning to be happy again. It never ends..."

"C'mon Rosemary, at least he's okay, could have been worse." I stare out the window full of gloom. "Think of this as the extended vacation you and Hugh always wanted but could never take. Use this time to your advantage. Instead of stressing so much, try to enjoy your time with him."

I'm not very receptive to his positive slant on the situation and fight hard to hold back my tears. *Vacation? This is a vacation? Emergency phone calls, seizures, tests, and doctors?*

The hospital calls twice in the short time I'm out. A neurologist wants to see Hugh right away. *Today.* I tell him I don't know how I will manage to get Hugh there. He's weak and has been feeling sick, but the doctor insists. Lee had to return to work. I don't have time to enlist help and it's pouring rain outside. I leave the girls a note and drive Hugh to St. Mary's hospital to meet this new doctor. He examines Hugh and schedules blood work, MRI and EEG labs. Then he informs us that Hugh's license is temporarily suspended for medical reasons—he will not be able to drive a car until he is seizure-free for a full six months. On our way out the door, Hugh slumps in resignation, too dopey and tired to be angry. He mumbles the one word he should be screaming, "Shit."

The medicine Hugh takes to control his seizures makes him lethargic and dazed, but we are told it is the one drug that is well-tested and usually prevents another seizure, so the doctor suggests he stay on it several weeks before switching to something else.

I write in my journal: *Spent the last two days driving the kids to school, Hugh to real estate class, girls to dance, doctors, store, dentist. Sit, sit, sit in the car, wait, wait, wait. Last night to LabCorp for blood work—sit, sit, sit, in doctor's office—wait, wait, wait.* My handwriting looks like that of a severely disturbed person.

My life exists in two places: the car and the waiting room, and if I'm not in one of those two places I'm on the phone, pressing 1 or zero for an operator. I have great difficulty scheduling an MRI and EEG for Hugh since he can only tolerate an open MRI or else he needs a sedative and the sedative screws up the EEG test. Then there's the complication that he has twenty-one screws in his head. I scramble around to find out if they are titanium screws or not, so the tests can be done. By the end of the day, I write an email to Kate:

What I need is a straight jacket, a tranquilizer and a month in the hospital, never mind the Bahamas. My Life is a F@!$#!!g Mess.*

She calls me the next morning, seriously worried about my mental state and reminds me again to take care of myself. I don't even know what that means anymore.

The rest of February is a waste. Hugh and I exist in a dismal funk. He's zoned out on anti-seizure meds and I'm just plain miserable. I'm thankful the girls are in school or dancing so they don't see a lot of us. Little by little, our friends nudge us out of the hole again.

The day before my forty-seventh birthday, the sun comes out to lift my dreary mood. Electra treats me to a full evening of drinks, dinner, dessert and girl-talk at four different places. On my birthday, March 12th, Peggy treats me to soup, salad and hot breadsticks for lunch and Hugh and the girls take me out to dinner. Our meal is followed by a reception at the Deep Run High School for Henrico county students who achieved top PSAT scores. Both Mary and Anna are recognized. *Okay, a step up,* I think. *At least he's sitting beside me this time.*

By St. Patrick's Day, Hugh comes alive again. He's seeing a neurologist who's weaning him on to an anti-seizure drug with fewer side effects. Now that he's less sedated, he takes an interest in exercise once more. He even takes the initiative to call someone about a possible part-time job as a financial planner. The job is on the south side of

Richmond, though, and since he can't drive, it's not workable.

While Hugh has more energy, there's not enough going on in his life to keep him busy. A call from Rick instantly cheers him up. He wants Hugh to go for a bike ride with him over the weekend, just around the neighborhood.

"Absolutely not, Hugh. Are you crazy or something?" I ask while biting my cuticle. He pushes my hand away from my mouth.

"Look Rosemary, I rode my bike every day for almost twenty years. I won't feel normal until I can ride a bike again. If it makes you happy to watch me sit in a chair...."

"Of course that doesn't make me happy, but you could really get hurt again. Why does it have to be a bike? Why can't you walk, or run, or play golf?"

"I want to ride again." His face is set in stone.

"Ugh!" I grunt. "I want you to live your life fully too..." Hugh surrounds me with one of his hugs. It's a losing battle. I'm uncomfortable with any talk of bikes, but when I look up at him and see his face so animated, it's reason enough to agree. "Okay, but please, please do not get hurt!"

The bike ride provides two full days of activities for Hugh. He digs around the garage, checking tire tubes and seats, reorganizing his gear, and anticipating the simple joy of riding again. Because I agreed, he hugs me every time our paths cross.

"A short neighborhood ride, I promise, nothing dangerous," he insists with a reassuring squeeze. All I can think is: *if he gets hurt again, it's my fault. It's my fault for not stopping him.*

Mary says to me later, "I can't believe you're going to let him do it, Mom!"

"It's who he is, Mary. Could you go through life without ever dancing again?"

"I wouldn't want to. But this is different."

"I know. I know! I just can't take this away from him," I say, hoping that I am not making a huge mistake.

On a warm Sunday afternoon, Rick and Hugh glide down the driveway on their favorite two-wheel mode of transportation. Hugh is tired. He had worked on his taxes with Lee in the morning, so he's dragging a bit from cognitive fatigue. Nevertheless, he's enthusiastic.

I sit out on the back deck with Rick's wife. "I hate that he wants to ride his bike again, Lara," I say. "When I tell him I don't want him to ride his bike or surf, he feels like he's being stripped of everything he loves. He's thinking he'll one day ride like he used to, but even this little bike ride with Rick is making my stomach churn. I don't know if I can live in this state of constant anxiety. I either make *him* miserable or make *myself* miserable. It's a lose lose situation."

I see Lara's sensible face soften with understanding. "Rick says he's going to take it really easy, very short. I know he'll be careful, Rosemary. If this had happened to Rick, he would want to ride again too. I don't know if I could handle it. I think I would be a nut case."

Looking through the ice water in my glass at the distorted image of the trees in my backyard, I admit, "I am a basket case. I see everything so differently now. You know what the hardest part is? We never used to tell each other what to do. That's all changed. I feel like I tell him all the time what to do next and what he can't do. We both feel stuck and resentful, and at the same time, we understand each other's point of view."

About an hour later, a frazzled looking Rick steps into the foyer and motions to me that the ride did not go well. Hugh is right behind him. He says nothing as he climbs the stairs to change his clothes, and clean up a scrape on his knee that he tries to hide. Rick tells me that Hugh fell off his bike twice during the ride and his balance was unstable. The thought that Hugh can no longer ride a bike strikes the very core of Rick. He knows Hugh as a man who was once more comfortable leaning into a fast corner on two wheels than he was walking. The realization hits Hugh even harder. He retreats to his chair.

Within a few days, he chalks it up to bad luck. He will work harder on improving his balance and try again to ride his bike in a few months. I take Hugh to the gym and work out with him a few days a week, or drop him there by himself. He seems more determined than ever to push himself physically. I even try jogging with him in the neighborhood, though I am the world's slowest runner. The memory in his rock hard legs returns, and he's quickly able to outrun my asthmatic lungs. As the wet month of March draws to a close, Hugh feels more alert and energetic. Optimism returns. He has not had a seizure in several weeks, and if he can just have a little patience he'll have his license back by the end of summer.

The phone rings on April 13th, a day I don't like to answer the phone. It's been one full year since his accident. Hugh picks it up. "Hey Michaelle," he says, and then glances over at me with a delighted look on his face. "She's calling to wish me Happy Anniversary!" Her call is quite a surprise considering he isn't even attending rehab at Health-South anymore. Hugh laughs into the phone with her and tells me afterward how she listed all his accomplishments. While somewhat embarrassed, his inward smile shines on his face. "She is a great therapist in more ways than one," I say.

As spring approaches, I put off my job search so there will be a driver in the family over the summer. The decision is liberating. The summer before had been completely lost to the injury. We decide to make this one count.

Hugh's twelve-month neuropsychological evaluation reveals that he has made significant gains on several tests. There are still lingering problems, but they are less severe than they had been—one was an impaired ability to learn, however, he took the Virginia real estate licensing test and recently passed, so we're not overly concerned about that one. More than ever, Hugh's continued progress leads me to believe that the brain's capacity to heal is unknown, and possibly unlimited. Hugh has shown an uncanny ability to overcome or compensate for many of his problems. As soon as a deficit is pointed out to him, he devises ways to improve. Now, he's determined to build his stamina and slowly reenter the workforce.

It's time to convert to COBRA at a huge personal expense to remain insured. We now feel the financial pinch that the last twelve months have forced upon us. Where is that insurance settlement? We're beginning to believe we'll be forced to go through with a court action. Regardless of what the insurance companies do, we have to pay the lawyer, doctor's bills, and other expenses as we go. I now see why there are so many banged-up old cars at rehab: no one can afford a decent one. Victims of accidents are often victims in many more ways than their physical injuries.

The last few weeks of March, we step up our therapy with Dr. Kreutzer to discuss how all these changes are affecting our lives and marriage. We have a tense discussion when Hugh expresses an interest in surfing. Until the seizures are under control, the doctor feels he should wait. I can see that look on Hugh's face, the one that says "Hmm, that's only one opinion." His strong will to continue in risky sports really irks me.

The weather is warming up and I want Hugh to be happy in the summer. It has always been his favorite time of year. For the first time I wish I had a big fat lazy husband who was content flipping burgers and fishing at the shoreline; at least maybe that way he'd stay alive! Nah, I immediately think, he'd manage to be an extreme fisherman rocking on some dinghy in the Atlantic trying to reel in a shark! I'll settle for the bike.

Chapter 40

Aloha Hugh,

I am sending you warm wishes and healing thoughts from beautiful Hawaii. It is a typical tropical day here today. The balmy trade winds are blowing gently through the palm trees and the sun is warm on my face. I hear the surf is small, but good for the boaters. We don't get to surf much now, but we still pay attention to the swell, old surfers never retire. We are in the barrel in spirit.

My positive thoughts and wishes for a complete recovery,
Nancy Tomlinson

-Rosemary's high school friend

One year out

Spring break arrives and our friends, Celie and Greg Florence (we call Greg "Flo" for short), offer us their oceanfront beach house for the week in the Outer Banks of North Carolina. We pack up the Explorer and I drive the family, using Hugh as my navigator. He knows the area well from numerous surf trips to Cape Hatteras when he was a teenager.

Dolphin's Retreat, as the house is named, sits on a grassy ocean dune in Southern Shores. The large two-story beach house sprouts a deck on every side encasing comfy padded chaise lounges and cushioned chairs designed for dreaming. The back deck overlooks a private access walkway to the ocean just beyond the outdoor shower, hot tub, and pool. On the main level, a window-lined family room, pastel-colored fabric sofas, and a table that seats eight are enhanced by a seaside motif. Pictures and statues of dolphins splash across walls and surfaces.

As I enter this sunlit haven, the weight of the past few months melts away. Bright light streams in warming me to the bone. Anna clicks on the nearest radio in the kitchen and grabs my hand away from the grocery bag I'm unpacking. "C'mon Mom, let's dance!" she shouts. Mary hears us from the front door, races up the steps and start jamming with us as Hugh watches with a calm smile. Mary calls out, "Dad, over here!" and motions him to join in the fun. Hugh crosses his arms over his chest, shakes his head 'No' and says, "You know I only slow dance." He steps out onto the high back deck overlooking the ocean and yells over the music, "Hey, there are dolphins out there!" Mary grabs a pair of binoculars she finds handily set by the glass sliding door. The dance party comes to an abrupt halt as we all squish through the doors and lean over the deck railing. Families of dolphins, leaping like a small welcoming party, perform graceful half moon jumps across the blue expanse of sparkling water. "Remember watching *Flipper* when we were kids?" I ask Hugh. He shakes his head nostalgically. "Isn't that on Nick at Night?" Anna asks.

The week passes by like a slow easy stroll. The day after we arrive, we drive south to explore. "I can't believe how many houses and stores there are now," Hugh says. "This was a barren stretch of road back when I used to surf here." The girls want lunch so we stop off at Capt'N Franks. Afterward we browse the Whalebone Surf Shop and check out The Pit for the surfing t-shirts Anna and Mary are hunting down. At night, we drive north and browse the shops in Duck, walking along the winding boardwalk outlining the sound. In one gift shop, Hugh spots me admiring a pair of iridescent blue earrings. "Here, buy those," he says tugging his wallet from his back pocket. At the register, I tell the sales lady, "I won't need a bag," as I slip on the earrings—my first real gift from Hugh since his accident.

On the beach, Hugh and I sit in the sand, but we don't go in the waves. They beckon Hugh like the curl of fingers calling him, but he resists. He had consulted Dr. Ward for that second opinion, and his answer was even more alarming than Dr. Kreutzer's. "Well, Hugh, people our age don't usually hurt their heads in the ocean, they usually break their necks. I don't recommend you swimming until your seizures are under control. But if you insist on going in, you should definitely wear a life jacket." That sealed it—Hugh won't be caught dead in a life jacket; he's a proud former ocean lifeguard. Our saving grace is that the water is ice cold and Hugh prefers to feel warm. The frigid tingling of the whitewash on his toes shoots up his leg like a warning that says 'not yet.' Hugh says, "Just being here is enough for now."

This is our first vacation in two years and we savor every second of it like licks off a favorite ice cream cone. Hugh feels intimately connected to the peace it provides. "Wouldn't it be just incredible to live in a place like this all the time?" he remarks to me while reclining in a lounge chair. As he gazes out over the dunes toward the sea, the look in his eyes intensifies. It's a look I've seen on his face many times before a bike race. In his mind, he is surfing. He's popping up on a short board turning left on a wave. Before his accident, Hugh was a proponent of visualization. When the girls were on swim team, he would coach them off the blocks. "See yourself gliding through the water; see yourself touching the wall," he would say just before the start.

My sister Peg shared a similar story with me once. She recalled Hugh teaching her to mountain bike. The rocky terrain and woods rattled her nerves as she wobbled forward. "Look where you want to go," Hugh called to her. "If you look at the tree, you'll hit the tree." She said she never forgot that lesson and that it has served her in more ways than one.

Hugh looks out at the water and sees where he wants to go.

A deep change penetrates everyone in our family on this trip. Our dark eyes brighten up with laughter. Sitting in high-backed canvas chairs along the shore, Hugh and I watch the girls dance in and out of the foaming water. High shrieks of laughter erupt and shivers ripple their backs as the waves hit their bare mid sections. Their slender arms shoot straight up as the shock of each icy wall of water breaks over their perfect teenage bodies. Later, in wetsuits, they paddle in. The neoprene provides some warmth, but their heads, feet, and fingers are exposed and numb. From the shore, we see shiny white heels rise and dip over the waves. Time spent in the water is short. Lips quiver and turn blue. The girls emerge hopping up and down, then race to the hot tub to let the jets massage their muscles into jelly.

As Hugh and I climb in and join them, we let out sighs of pleasure. Every one of our senses come alive: we feel the hot water pulsing our skin, we hear the sound of the waves rolling and crashing, we see white billowing clouds against blue sky, and we taste the salt-soaked air. Hugh can no longer smell the salt air. "I think that's the smell I miss the most," he confesses. "That, and brownies baking."

Each day that week, we walk further and further to destinations that Hugh marks along the way. "Today we'll make it to the yellow beach house. Tomorrow we'll make it to that Jolly Roger flag way over there!" We know he has cheated death, and for the first time since his accident, we're really enjoying life again.

Together, we rediscover something in ourselves that has been missing for a very long time: playfulness. I thought it had disappeared forever. Its return feels like the first glimpse of the sun's rays after a long stretch of stormy weather. We arrive home just before Easter, the season of rebirth and renewal, where all things are possible.

Chapter 41

Year Two
Early May- Early July

On a busy morning in mid May, I have to go out while the girls are in school. Hugh stays in bed upstairs to watch a bike race on television. Before I leave, I ask him to answer the phone if it rings because I'm expecting a call. When I arrive home, Hugh calls me upstairs.

"Are you feeling okay?" I ask.

"Not really," he says. "I jumped up when the phone rang and rushed to answer it in my office. I got lightheaded, and leaned on the credenza to talk. When I tried to go back to the bedroom, I landed on the floor face down."

"Did you hurt yourself?"

"I don't think so. But I don't know if I fell, fainted or had a seizure. I felt funny. Strange. What should we do?"

"I have to call the doctor, Hugh." His face droops.

"I know," he says. We both know what this means. But it's better than risking another seizure. We see the neurologist immediately. To be on the safe side, the doctor tacks on six more months of driving restriction, pushing the date up to November. Though disappointed, we are almost immune to bad news by now so we just shrug and drive home, the news somewhat expected.

Hugh's schedule is light. He makes a point of working out physically every day, but out of boredom, he watches too much television. It never fails to amaze me when I see him in his recliner reacting to jokes on "Home Improvement." His new lighter personality enjoys sitcoms, and it's nice to see him laugh, but I often wonder: *Who is this man sitting in my living room?*

The girls finish the school year. Mary joins swim team, Anna joins the high school dance team that has a summer camp, and both girls attend several dance workshops at Shuffles. After seeing Hugh at the beach, I call a friend of mine, Jason Blake, to see if he can work with Hugh in the water. Jason, a former NOVA swimmer and swim coach, works at American Family Fitness as a personal trainer. He tells me he's eager to work with Hugh and will research brain injury before meeting us for the first time at the indoor pool in the gym.

At their first session, Hugh enters the pool area from the locker room clad in a baggy swimsuit that hangs on his now skinny hips. Jason instructs him to get into the lap pool using the ladder. "Is it cold?" Hugh asks.

"You'll get used to it," Jason replies. Hugh gingerly enters the water at the low end—about waist deep—and within seconds he is visibly shivering. Jason hands him a pair of goggles to put on. The rubber straps make Hugh's ears stick out. He looks vulnerable, like a ten-year-old boy, but Jason says, "Okay now, let me see your stroke. Swim to the end of the pool." Hugh begins to swim the front crawl; his stroke is choppy and slow. Jason looks at me approvingly and says, "We'll need to work on that left rotator cuff. He just needs some practice and strength training." Hugh makes it to the end of the pool, shaking. "It's too cold," he says through chattering teeth.

"You need to swim more to warm up. Good job, Hugh. Your left shoulder is tight but it looks like we can work on that and improve your range of motion," Jason replies. As chilly as Hugh is, he swims back to us and is done for the day. From this point on, Jason takes over. Each week, he picks Hugh up at the house, works out with him at the gym, and drops him home. Twenty-five years his junior, with a Masters degree in Sports Leadership, Jason is the perfect medicine for Hugh. He is fit, intelligent, and energetic. He pushes Hugh to his limit in a demanding, customized workout designed to improve strength, balance, and brain function. Hugh eats it all up and begs for more. These workout sessions do more for him than improve his strength, co-ordination, and muscle tone, they improve his confidence and stamina as well.

In the balmy month of June, and before the heat oppressive height of the season, Hugh runs almost daily and takes care of the yard. I begin classes at the University of Richmond to finish my degree in Human Resource Management. I want to be prepared for a full-time job if Hugh can't return to a position that has health benefits. I have no idea what I will do with my small home-based résumé writing business, but it sure doesn't generate enough cash for a busy family of four. The court case is paramount now. It looms ahead in a matter of weeks. Liz begins calling almost daily for information to prepare for the trial.

As I work on a research paper for my first class, prepare résumés for clients, drive the girls to all their activities, and keep up the housework I can fit in between all the rest, I feel drained and overextended. Stacks of papers and tasks like tracking down one thing or another for the impending court case or trying to straighten out some bill or insurance problem always sidetrack me. The cars need inspections and we have planned a trip to visit family in New York. I know this insanity will be temporary, so I tell myself to just get through it. My back aches and my stomach itches. I have no idea what is wrong with me, but I keep up the schedule.

July first is our twenty-fifth wedding anniversary. We celebrate at home with a big dinner. Hugh's parents and my brother, John, and his family join us as they pass through Richmond from their home in Atlanta, Georgia. As I reach up to get a wine glass from the cupboard, my sister-in-law, Susan, asks, "What's that on your back?"

"I have no idea. I think some weird bug got into my shirt or something and bit me all over. It's been itching for days. It's on my stomach too."

"Rosemary, let me see that." She looks closely and carefully in her science-teacher way, lifting my shirt a little for a serious inspection. After a moment, she calls my brother over to have a look. "Would you two stop," I whine while trying to take care of dishes in the kitchen as they pull my shirt, and talk about the redness.

"That's not bug bites. You need to see the doctor," John says, looking concerned.

"I don't have time to see a doctor," I say flatly. "I'm driving everyone to New York in two days so I can relax a little by Mom and Dad's pool, and I wouldn't miss that for the world."

"You'd better make time, Rosemary. That looks nasty! You have to take care of yourself too," Susan chimes in. They both make me promise to check it out.

The following morning, my back burns, so I call the doctor. He takes one look at it and says, "Classic case of shingles, likely caused by stress." He says it will go away on its own but will take some time. If we had caught it sooner, he might have been able to give me medicine, but it won't work now. "Try to get some rest and call me if it gets any worse," he instructs.

It is not as if I have time to be sick, so after my night class at seven-thirty, I pick Anna up from the dance studio. We drive to join Hugh and Mary at a swim meet. Clouds are gathering quickly and soon the rain starts pouring in sheets; the heavy scent of mossy mold and chlorine hovers over the entire pool area. "That pool smells so strong," I remark to Hugh, who promptly answers, "I wouldn't know." He gives me a husbandly smile when I mumble an apology. We gather and huddle under a tarp by the pool hearing the drum of water beating on canvas until after eleven p.m. when the final ribbon is slapped and soggy towels are gathered at the end of the swim meet.

By the time we arrive home, my right side and back are on fire. I coat the rash with thick pink lotion making it looks like the skin of an old cracked baby doll. The dark red of the shingles shows right through the thick pink goo that dries to a powdery cake. Without even speaking, everyone trudges to bed, exhausted. Early the following morning, we pack the car and I drive the seven hours to my parent's house in East Northport, New York while my three passengers doze on and off.

On arrival, my mother remarks that I look tired. As we sit out under the birch trees in the shade, I explain to her what the doctor told me: "Hugh has never been sure if he had the chickenpox and I might be contagious to him. So, I need to be careful not to let him touch my rash…and it's our anniversary trip!" I lift up my shirt to show her. My mother lets out a gasp, then a deep sigh.

"Don't worry, Mom, I packed my long pajama pants and will keep them pulled up to my waist! So much for romance!" I say. She laughs, and says, "Leave it to you to think of THAT!" We both raise our eyebrows and smile. My mother says, "Oh honey, will it ever end? At least you can laugh."

This week gives us all time to relax and think. While the girls play badminton with Hugh, I sit on a chaise lounge and reflect. Nancy Foley had been right. Trying to keep all the pieces of my life together without counseling would work for only so long. After that, there would be physical consequences. The strain is beginning to show outwardly. I have been thinking about the question that Nancy repeatedly asked me, "What are you really feeling, Rosemary?" The truth is: I don't allow time to feel. I fill up every moment of every day with work and activity and take a sleeping pill if I can't sleep at night so I cannot possibly feel anything. But lately, the feelings come anyway…they come and they come and they come.

I am a dangling eyehook caught on the fragile thread of a well-worn garment. If I let go, all will fall away. My place in this family is central. Hugh has always represented the hero in our family, but I am the compass and barometer, the tone, pitch, and mood. I am the pulse and the heart of my family and like it or not, when I'm miserable, everyone is miserable. And so I push, and smile, and cajole, and I cry in private.

Hugh created our lifestyle through his hard work. He happily showered us all with gifts and excitement: a nice home, cars, vacations, and the perks of good living. He has also been the provider of glorious moments for the girls: soaring down the block with no hands on a bicycle; riding a wave on a surfboard for the first time. I provide stability, lessons, and comfort. I work behind the scenes and draw back the curtain that showcases my family's amazing resilience. I am the organizer, the soother, and the appeaser.

I am the mother and I'm falling apart.

I don't know myself anymore. Try as I might to live in the 'now,' the past year has swallowed me whole. It has robbed my natural joyous nature, and left me feeling brittle and uncertain.

Questions and troubling thoughts flood my mind. They keep me up nights and leak into my brain all day. Hugh has changed and so has our life together. Was this accident meant to change me? How can I let it change me for the better rather than consume me, frighten me, or draw me into a funnel of fear, always thinking about what might happen next? I've become an annoying pest, even to myself. I hear myself speak as if I'm hearing a neurotic stranger constantly telling everyone to be careful, constantly needing reassurance. Do you have your cell phone? Did you take your pills? Are you too tired to drive?

How do I return to living each day without imagining accidents? Why can't I go about my day without fearing the worst, reciting endless prayers for protection, wanting to help everyone, wanting to give back so much I can't handle all the giving back, taking bad news personally, as if it's happening to me, wanting to make it all better for everyone, wanting to make it all go away?

How do I go back to life as a plain and simple person again? Or should I?

Can I let the repercussions of Hugh's accident drench into me without drowning? Something's eating me alive, gnawing at me: the realization that I may die suddenly, without warning, or worse, that others I love will die before me. I feel threatened on a level so close it's heart-stopping. I once felt so connected and safe in the world, but now I know that our connections can't save us. We are alone in our individual thoughts, passage, and experience. We are ultimately alone in our grief. We must dissect our own truth, examine it, make sense of it, and accept it.

So we can let go of it.

Feelings of grief, loss, fear, and the unknown plunge me into waking blackouts, moments so intense I stop breathing. The inevitable is the eventual separation through death, a permanent leaving, a physical departure, yet I know there is a spiritual presence; I felt the strength of others reaching out to me in the days and weeks following Hugh's accident like a psychic force. Will I ever find solid comfort in that? Will I ever find peace?

The answer hangs in the distance among a billion other questions. It's yes with hard work. It's yes with suffering. It's yes worth getting to because the journey is so long and arduous. But the answer is yes.

When we get home, I finally call a counselor and ask her for help.

Chapter 42

Note to self: Next vanity plate "HuprDuprMan"

Year two
Late July 2003-November 2003

I answer the phone and hear the jubilant voice of our lawyer, Liz. "Darlin, I have good news, but I have to tell my client first. Put Hugh on." I stand nearby shifting from one foot to the other while he whispers, "Uh huh" into the phone before signing off with, "Will do! Thanks for everything."

"Well?" I say as he slowly hangs up the phone.

"We don't have to go to court. We got a settlement offer," he says. I fall into a celebratory hug.

Common sense tells me it's time to put the past in perspective and move forward, despite the fact that Hugh's TBI will always be misunderstood by the vast majority of people going about their day-to-day business. There will be long term effects and medication required for years to come. "I guess it's time to move on," Hugh says. "But where? What's my goal now?" He is quiet and pensive for a day or two.

The black pavement of the road emanates heat left over from the hot August sun as we take our usual walk up to Broad Street in the evening. I can see that more than the heat is weighing Hugh down. "We got the settlement, so what's on your mind?" I ask.

Slowing his pace, he says, "I don't feel like an athlete anymore."

I stop him. "Oh yes you are! After thirty years of being an athlete, you are not an athlete because of *what* you can *do,* but because of *who* you are: a team player, someone who never quits, who strives to be his personal best, and who believes in fair play. You do all these things, Hugh. You always have." He mulls this over but seems only half convinced.

"There's nothing to wake up for in the morning," he says. "Well, you and the girls..." he mutters.

"I know what you mean. We'll figure something out," I say. "For now, let's celebrate that we won't go bankrupt, and that we never have to think about that awful woman who hit you again." After our walk, we indulge in big bowls of ice cream at home.

A day or two later, a friend stops by to say hello. She tells me about an organization that helps people start or grow their small businesses. Many of the volunteer coaches are retired executives. As she talks to me about it, I can't help but think this is custom made for Hugh, so I venture, "Terry, would you talk to Hugh about this?" She agrees, and before you know it, she's picking Hugh up and taking him along with her to the meetings where he works on a few projects with new business owners. This volunteer job refines his computer skills as he becomes more limber in his typing and more proficient navigating the Internet.

When September rolls around, Hugh asks Kevin if he'll take him on a bike ride. It's an activity he is determined to master again. They make a date for Saturday morning.

I make sure to give Hugh a kiss before he goes and fight the urge to say, "Be careful" a hundred times. Reading my face, Kevin says, "Rosemary, believe me, I'll be careful as hell out there, because I know I have to answer to you if anything happens!" They load the bikes onto the Explorer and Kevin drives Hugh to West Creek, where the traffic is light and the terrain perfect for a leisurely ride.

Two hours later they return. "Your husband is a pro," announces Kevin. "He managed the bike around potholes and all!"

Later I ask Hugh, "How does it feel to be back on the bike?"

He thinks for a moment. "It was hard, it took all my concentration, but I think if I practice it will become second nature." I feel my jaw tighten at the thought of him on a bike, but I also recognize my own physical symptoms and concentrate on stopping them.

I inwardly repeat the mantra I discussed with my counselor. *Hugh is not asking me to let him do dangerous things; he wants to ride a bike. Many people ride bikes and don't get hurt.* I try to look happy for him.

Over the next few weeks Hugh's determination soars to an all time high as he masters riding again. His athletic mindset to ignore limits and push ahead pays off. Lifting weights and cross training in the gym benefits him cognitively as well as physically. As he becomes stronger, his balance and endurance improve to the point where he can join his old group rides. I still feel a familiar chill of dread when he's on the bike. His eager face is the only thing that keeps me from begging him not to go.

The disturbing flashbacks I imagine of Hugh's accident are a continuing problem for me. I see a new LCSW who helps me delve into my own feelings about the past seventeen months. She tells me I'm exhibiting symptoms of hyper-vigilance, a state in which I'm always on the lookout to ensure that everyone is safe. My symptoms are sleeplessness, anxiety, a tendency to want to overprotect my family, and my fear of car accidents or driving in bad weather. This state of mind was brought on by post-traumatic stress because of the severity and duration of Hugh's injury. Through a series of discussions and with the help of a relaxation tape, I am beginning to feel better and sleep more soundly. Hugh is considerate and understanding.

"Hon, look, just tell me what you want me to do to make you feel better and I'll do it," he offers. "Just don't say I can't ride at all." He agrees to a few ground rules like riding only with other people and avoiding areas with traffic.

Early one evening, I see him toweling off after a shower. "The days feel longer and longer. I never thought I'd say this, but I wish I had a real job," he says. Volunteering and looking after his small real estate holdings with Lee take up only a few hours each week. "Look, it's five-thirty and I have nothing to do—nothing on the calendar tomorrow. It's weird."

Ever since the night I had asked Lee to see if he thought Hugh might be ready for work, he has come over periodically to quietly evaluate Hugh's progress as it pertains to an executive position in accounting and finance. One evening, Hugh and Lee spend a few hours in Hugh's upstairs office. Afterward, Lee sneaks up behind me in the kitchen with a smile on his face and whispers, "He's ready."

Within a week, over dinner in a restaurant, Lee introduces Hugh to the president of a local engineering company. When Hugh arrives home, he tells me about the dinner. "Lee's friend, George, is a nice guy. He's having some accounting issues in his company, so I gave him a few suggestions and he seemed receptive." Later in the week, Hugh corresponds with George and after a few notes back and forth, he begins consulting for him part-time in September of 2003. "I don't care about the money. It's just so great to feel useful again," Hugh says.

Working out of our home offices, we both feel more productive. Hugh has organized his office upstairs. I write résumés at my desk downstairs and check my email frequently. There is usually one from Hugh asking what's for dinner or some other question. Each note feels like a triumph. Our conversations turn to business topics at the lunch table. I share the business books I'm reading at the University of Richmond with Hugh and he devours them.

In mid-November, Hugh is once again granted the right to drive. He spends nearly the entire day running errands in the car. "Need anything at the store?" he asks.

"Not since you went an hour ago," I answer. He's also taking correspondence courses to catch up on continuing education credits so he can be re-certified as a CPA. He studies with a vengeance. "I don't know why I used to complain about going to work. I would do anything now to have my old job back," he tells me.

The issue of financial security comes up. What if he does not succeed in his job? It has already happened once. I make a few calls and discover that there is a nine-month trial period where Hugh can try to work full-time and if it doesn't work out, he can revert to his disability status. With that cushion in place, he decides it's time to take the plunge.

I write Hugh a résumé—the most important résumé of my career—and the only person who receives it is George. Hugh takes online tests and aces his interview at the engineering company as George engages in a formal search for his top financial executive.

One month shy of the two-year anniversary of his accident, Hugh attains his goal. He's a Chief Financial Officer. Patty King calls soon after we get the news. "Hugh is a walking miracle, Rosemary," she says. I think of the strange way Hugh's accident flipped our roles these past two years, how I called on the lessons Hugh had taught me as I watched him coach people in the past. And though these long months were grueling, like running a marathon with someone riding-piggy back and the finish line moving every time you draw near, it was my way of learning that life has no finish line. In fact, the racecourse can detour dramatically at any moment, so we better not become too attached to the familiar footpath.

With Hugh out at the office and the girls halfway through high school, I'm energized by the long list of things I want to achieve because I feel intensely alive again. I add extra classes to finish the degree I put on hold many years ago, reconnect with friends, go out to lunch, and read stories that help me forget to stress. And the journal I began in the emergency room nearly two years ago continues to serve me. Writing, more than anything, clears out my dusty mind. It has helped me find meaning and recognize progress—the pebbles of progress that have formed the foundation of our new life.

Epilogue

Outer Banks, NC - Summer, 2008
Six years after accident

Hugh checks surfline.com on Friday night before we pack the car and drive from Richmond to the Outer Banks of North Carolina to spend the week—three hours door to door. "It's flat," he reports sadly. With a sudden change of heart he smiles and adds, "But I'll have my girls. I'll just ride the long board." These few beach days are special because they will be our only time together as a family all summer. Anna and Mary are both home for a short break at the end of their college semesters; they'll both return to New York for the summer.

We pull into the parking lot and unload coolers of food and supplies for a few days of beach living. Our small condo in Dare County—I can't get over the name of our new county—looks out on Kitty Hawk Bay, yet we are only a mile from the ocean. After spending many weekends visiting the outer banks, Hugh finally convinced me that we should own a small place there. It wasn't easy. "Can we afford it?" I kept asking.

"Can we afford not to?" he said. "I want to enjoy the ocean while I still can, not when I'm old and sick. We've always been sensible, so we'll manage. Hell, we've earned it."

We closed on our two-bedroom retreat in November 2005. Like newlyweds, we blasted the radio and painted with the windows open in winter. We took hot showers and made love in the afternoon on the living room floor by the fireplace.

On this Saturday morning in June, Hugh is the first one up. He loads the boards on top of the car while I pack a picnic. "I think Dad's ready, girls, better hurry up," I say to Mary and Anna as they finish their toast. We're heading out for a surf safari in search of any wave large enough to ride. In the Ford Freestyle, my head leans against the edge of the open window as the wind whips my hair on the stretch of road leading south toward Cape Hatteras. The girls sit together in the back smelling of coconut sunscreen.

"Hey, I heard they made a movie using the house at Rodanthe," Anna says as we approach the weather-beaten structure that juts out of nowhere like an ancient castle. The ocean laps at the exposed foundation making me think of Atlantis. As my mind spirals into dreaded global warming scenarios and storm surges that could bury the outer banks completely, Hugh is grounded in the present. "I just hope people don't stalk the place now…a great surf break will turn into a tourist spot," he jokes. "Let's check out the swell," he adds pulling the car over to the side of the road. He jumps out, crosses Highway 12 and runs up and over the high dune with the girls and me at his heels. "Not much going on. What do you think?" he asks.

"I say we head south," Anna says.

"Okay, back in the car," Hugh says.

By the time we arrive at Hatteras the sun is hot. The girls set out beach towels and lie in the sand. Hugh can barely wait to get in the water. After paddling out, he bobs patiently, watching for the best set before taking off on a wave. I think of the poster we saw in a surf shop that read, "The Ocean is My Temple." Hugh pointed to it and said, "That's my religion, right there." I know he's right. Since his accident, he's been more drawn to the ocean than ever. I often wonder if he was hypnotized in the ICU when I kept telling him he was warm at the ocean as he slept under an ice blanket in a coma. I've seen him swim and surf for hours and emerge luminescent as though baptized, body and soul.

I walk along the shore toward the lighthouse writing stories in my head. Hugh can't understand why I like to write. He's taking evening classes for his MBA and hates writing papers. My mother tells him, "Her words are your waves."

"Give me a spreadsheet any day," he says.

With little fanfare, I closed Résumés Worth Reading in February. I graduated from the University of Richmond in May and met with the director of the Brain Injury Association of Virginia to map out some volunteer work for the summer.

Mary sneaks up behind me, "Anna's in the water with Dad. Can I walk with you?" she asks. I nod to her. We gather shells along the way that I hold in my baseball cap. Beach chairs and umbrellas disappear as we stroll away from the crowded part of the shore.

"I only have one week to spend at the beach this summer," Mary laments.

"Yeah, but you will be done with the program in May. It went so fast," I say.

"It did. I can't believe you guys let me leave college and go to AMDA in New York. I really appreciate it, Mom. It's hard, but I love it."

"You know, Mary, I think I realized that your getting an academic degree was *my* dream, not yours. Musical theater is your passion, like writing is mine. Dad and I are just glad you're happy. It took guts to do what you did." She tilts her head affectionately so it touches my shoulder as we walk. As an afterthought I ask, "Are you and Anna coming to Celie and Flo's for dinner tonight?"

"Does Flo cook for you *every* Saturday night?" she asks.

"Pretty much," I smile. "It works for us and he seems to enjoy it. We call it Chez Flo's."

"I think Anna made plans for us to go to a party, so don't count on us, but tell them we say 'hi.'" We turn around and start back to our spot by the jetty where Hugh and Anna are surfing. After a picnic of peanut butter and jelly sandwiches, Mary decides to join them in the water.

From my beach chair, I watch Hugh balance on a wave. He has worked steadily as a Chief Financial Officer for the past four years, first for George, and then moving to a larger company. He's been off antidepressants for years now, and his stamina far exceeds my own. He never wants to sleep. After he worked a year, I surprised him with a gift: a trip to Australia to surf with his boyhood best friend. While there, he surfed inside the barrel of a wave, an amazing accomplishment for anyone to achieve, no less an individual who had once lost all balance and coordination.

Dr. Kreutzer says Hugh is by far the best TBI recovery he has ever seen, and he has seen over 5,000 patients. For everyone else, the accident is over. It happened long ago, and it's done. Hugh recovered. For me, it's never over. I still fight anxiety and fear, but I'm also full of gratitude and joy for the way things turned out. I'm fully aware that the outcome is not this positive for most brain injury survivors, and I think about those less fortunate every day.

I look out at the ocean, my hand shielding my eyes from the glare, and find my three favorite people in the lineup. I can't help but admire them for finding the surface after such a deep plunge into murky unknown depths. Anna rides a leisurely wave almost to the shore before stepping off her board. She hops over the whitewater as if there are hot coals underfoot. Curly tendrils drip water as she leans forward to pull the Velcro of her ankle leash. I walk over. "Are you disappointed that the waves are small today?" I ask.

"Nah! Dad is having a blast, she says with a sunny smile. "It's all good."

CPSIA information can be obtained at www.ICGtesting.com
Printed in the USA
BVOW081057250911

272078BV00007B/5/P

9 781432 773250